T0266525

The Modern Salad

The Modern Salad

INNOVATIVE NEW AMERICAN AND INTERNATIONAL RECIPES
INSPIRED BY BURMA'S ICONIC TEA LEAF SALAD

ELIZABETH HOWES

ULYSSES PRESS

Text copyright © 2016 Elizabeth Howes. Photographs copyright © 2016 Kimberley Hasselbrink except as noted below. Design and concept copyright © 2016 Ulysses Press and its licensors. All rights reserved. Any unauthorized duplication in whole or in part or dissemination of this edition by any means (including but not limited to photocopying, electronic devices, digital versions, and the internet) will be prosecuted to the fullest extent of the law.

Published in the United States by:
Ulysses Press
P.O. Box 3440
Berkeley, CA 94703
www.ulyssespress.com

ISBN: 978-1-64604-232-6
Library of Congress Control Number: 2015952118

Printed in the United States
10 9 8 7 6 5 4 3 2 1

Acquisitions editor: Keith Riegert
Project editor: Alice Riegert
Managing editor: Claire Chun
Editor: Susan Lang
Proofreader: Kate St. Clair
Front cover and interior design: Ashley Prine
Layout: whatdesign @ whatweb.com
Photography: © Kimberley Hasselbrink except pages viii, 2, 3, 93, 100, 102 © Marion Montgomery; pages 4, 5, 6
    © Amy Iftekhar; pages 81, 83 © Elizabeth Howes
Food styling: Elizabeth Howes and Kimberley Hasselbrink

IMPORTANT NOTE TO READERS: This book is independently authored and published and no sponsorship or endorsement of this book by, and no affiliation with, any trademarked brands or other products mentioned within is claimed or suggested. All trademarks that appear in this book belong to their respective owners and are used here for informational purposes only. The authors and publisher encourage readers to patronize the quality brands and products mentioned in this book.

FOR FLETCHER

May you have the curiosity and courage to fearlessly follow the pull toward what you truly love. Your presence in my life is a daily reminder to live the same way. This book is for you. Thank you for being my master tester, source of infinite laughter, most honest critic, and invaluable teacher of life. My table—and my heart—will always be yours, sweet boy.

Contents

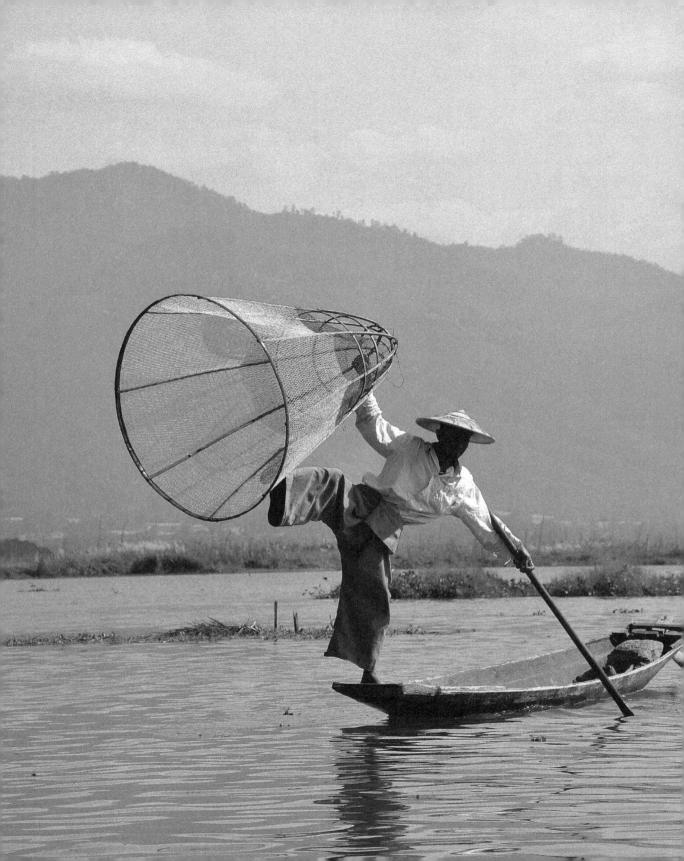

Note from the Author

Food has equated to happiness my entire life. From the time I was very young, the kitchen became my sanctuary, my refuge. My parents loved to cook and entertain, so the kitchen was quickly understood as a place of social agreement, kinship, and, for me, internal stability. No matter what was going on around me, this one room, whether I lived in a 500-square-foot studio in San Francisco or cooked in a client's 5,000-square-foot estate in Napa, was home.

This book is not about superfoods, despite the fact that I have incorporated many. It's not necessarily about achieving perfect health, or even about eating in the cleanest way possible. These elements are both included and important, however. The core of this book is about reinvention and the transformative power of exhilarating whole food.

By design, the salads in this book are uncommon. They're complex, and intense. And full of unexpected contradictions of flavor and texture that, I believe, only a few types of food can truly offer: tart and sweet; salty and bitter; crunchy and tender; spicy and cool; fresh and cooked.

Striking that powerful balance, and coming up with innovative, modern combinations that excite, was my goal in developing these recipes. To me, the magic of cooking lies in those contradictions, in these unexpected discoveries. This collection of recipes—brimming with fresh vegetables, fruits, spices, herbs, teas, roots, nuts, seeds, and ferments—inspires me. Not only because they are mine, but because they're brought to life from one iconic dish that people often describe as thrilling, addictive, and unlike anything they have ever tasted: the Burmese tea leaf salad.

My hope is that you'll find thrill and inspiration within these pages, too.

The Illustrious Story of the Tea Leaf Salad

Before Burma officially became Myanmar in 1989, this beloved salad was reserved for royalty, served only during special occasions because of the prized ingredients and compelling presentation. Today, this salad, called lahpet ("green tea") thoke ("to blend by hand") is enjoyed by many. From the moment it arrives at the table, it's a sensual and exhilarating experience. The grassy, sour, fermented green tea leaves form the acclaimed epicenter and are what makes this salad unforgettable. When the leaves are tossed, they infuse the entire dish with a bracing, acidic brightness.

Other unique ingredients also breathe life and balance into this fascinating salad. Sun-dried, briny ground shrimp, called bazun-chauk, provide a source of protein and bring forth the coveted savory umami flavor. Fried beans or peas supply an alluring crunch and pop that makes eating this salad such a lively experience. Then there are the fried slivers of crunchy garlic, and the oil they slowly infused, along with bright citrus and ginger that dance across the palate. Nutty seeds, toasted peanuts, and fresh tomatoes are also part of the extensive ingredient list. Arranged artfully and with precision in a deconstructed format, this salad is typically tossed tableside, where the slightly damp, tangy leaves permeate every inch of the salad. The end result is crunchy and chewy, bright and earthy, salty and tart, ultra-fresh, and irrefutably addictive.

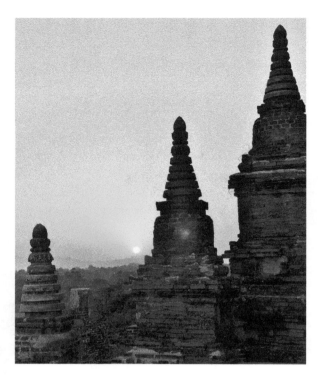

One of the national dishes of Myanmar, this salad is typically offered at the end of a meal because the fermented leaves are believed to be an effective digestive aid. During some of the most tumultuous times the Burmese people have endured, the tea leaf salad served as a symbolic peace offering and unspoken resolution of disputes. Today, it often graces the table at celebratory occasions such as weddings and religious ceremonies, and has become a popular street food. It is either arranged deconstructed in compartmentalized plates, allowing carte blanche to eat in any desired sequence, or is vigorously tossed together with bare hands before serving. It has been said that students also rely on this acclaimed dish during final exams for the stimulant zing it offers.

A SENSE OF PLACE

Despite the fact that the people of Myanmar create such riveting food, they have long been a culture trying to find its place in the world. There's a relentless dichotomy of positive and negative, shadow and light. Military rule, war, ethnic insurgencies, and isolation are part of their history, and this hardship is ingrained in them. Still, they possess the constant ability to reinvent. Their relationship with food, and the ritual of gathering around a table to cultivate community, serves as a sanctuary from daily strife. It is the simple rhythm of living, like cooking and eating, while enduring loss, displacement, and immense heartache, that has the ability to create a richness in place, in home. And that feeling is internally constructed and cannot be lost.

In her book, *The Art of Eating*, M.F.K. Fisher eloquently expanded upon this theory:

> I believe that one of the most dignified ways we are capable of, to assert and then reassert our dignity in the face of poverty and war's fears and pains, is to nourish ourselves with all possible skill, delicacy, and ever-increasing enjoyment. And with our gastronomical growth will come, inevitably, knowledge and perception of a hundred other things, but mainly ourselves. Then Fate, even tangled as it is with cold wars as well as hot, cannot harm us.

A COLLISION OF CUISINES

Nestled between China, India, Thailand, and Laos, Myanmar is the largest country in mainland Southeast Asia. The size of Texas, it is divided into seven states and seven divisions. Because Myanmar sits at a cultural crossroads, the cuisine has undergone its own reinvention and is the sum of many regional parts. Samosas (fried or baked pastries with savory fillings), curries, naan bread, and many spices were adopted from Indian cuisine. Complex and strong Thai aromatics, including some elements of fiery heat, also permeate the cuisine of Myanmar. And the Chinese influence shows up in soy sauce, wok techniques, and various noodle dishes. Finally, sticky rice powder, with its characteristic toasted flavor and unique texture, and larb, a finely chopped, deeply flavored meat salad, undoubtedly found their way to Myanmar by way of Lao cuisine.

Similarly, the various forms of tea consumption can be traced back thousands of years across these particular cultures.

TEA AND TERROIR

Native to Myanmar, tea grows wild all over the rolling, lush hills and is also meticulously grown and harvested by hand. The best is set aside for fermenting while the remainder is dried and made into tea for consumption. The first and most prized (first flush) harvest is usually in May and June, before the monsoons hit, but harvest often extends all the way to October.

To achieve maximum flavor, tea cultivation is not rushed. Three years is considered optimal to obtain a crop. Tea seeds are so fundamental to the culture that they are carried when people move from one settlement to another, and dried or fermented tea is a customary gift for visitors.

Tea consumption is a way of life in Myanmar. Teahouses, a legacy of the British colonial period, are popular hangouts. Buddhist monks sip the warm, calming brew throughout the day. Production is also sacred, remaining artisanal, with green and black tea as the primary commodities. Because of the strong cultural connection to tea, significant care goes into growing the crop.

As is true of the famous wine-growing regions of the world, the nuanced flavors of tea from this region are not happenstance. The environmental characteristics—the terroir—greatly affect the tea's character. Interactions between plant, climate, soil, altitude, sun exposure, and precipitation all come into play. Even less calculable are cultural and human factors. Warm and welcoming, the Burmese people center their lives around community and the rich land on which they thrive physically and economically.

THE SACRED ART OF TEA FERMENTATION

Fermenting, or pickling, tea is considered an art form and is typically carried out by the Palaung, the oldest tribe living in the largest state in Myanmar, Shan State. Women still wear traditional attire, including thick

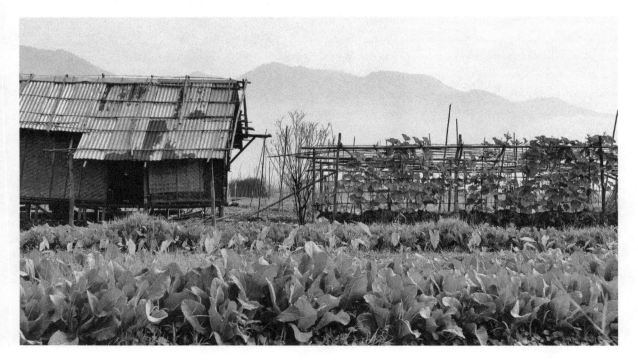

silver hoops around the waist to ward off evil spirits, jewel-toned velvet jackets, cloth leggings, and colorful bands composed as headdresses. These people are famous for the tea they grow and cure.

Palaung tea is cultivated on high-altitude (greater than 6,000 feet) plantations, where the leaves are intentionally grown at a slow rate. While the yields are lower and the terrain more treacherous, these plants are given time to develop deep, complex flavor. Very young leaves are harvested, steamed, rolled by hand, and sun-dried to make traditional green tea for drinking.

To create fermented green tea, a more complicated and sacred process is followed. Once the verdant leaves are harvested, they are gently steamed for about an hour, and then laid out on banana leaves or bamboo mats and mashed by hand. The leaves are then densely packed into baskets or bamboo vats, heavily weighted to expel any excess air, and buried in pits. They're left to ferment for a couple months, even up to a year. The longer fermentation process is often optimal as it creates intense flavor. The finished product is described as "an explosion of flavor" in Sandor Katz's book *The Art of Fermentation*.

Fermented tea leaves are slowly making their way to the West. Strict hygiene standards are finally being imposed for the fermentation and export process. These standards are providing tea farmers with international visibility, credibility, and greater income potential thanks to a broader market in which to offer the product they assiduously create.

THE STAYING POWER OF MODERN MYANMAR

Myanmar is a land full of more glowing golden temples and pagodas than anywhere else on earth. In the midst of ongoing turmoil, light and a spirit of reinvention still exist. The people are warm and gracious despite the endless struggle they've endured. There's an indestructible inner peace among the ruin. In a Nobel Lecture, the fourteenth Dalai Lama shared the following:

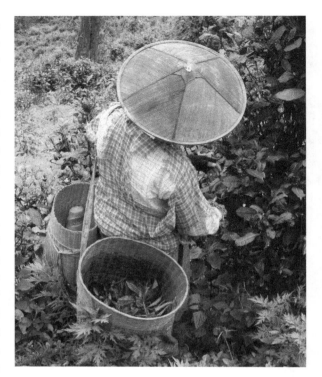

Inner peace is the key: if you have inner peace, the external problems do not affect your deep sense of peace and tranquility. In that state of mind, you can deal with situations with calmness and reason, while keeping your inner happiness. That is very important. Without this inner peace, no matter how comfortable your life is materially, you may still be worried, disturbed or unhappy because of circumstances.

This internal resiliency and strong value system have prepared Myanmar to move from severe constriction to astounding expansion. Now home to luxury hotels, modern agricultural practices—including wine production and organic food certification—and niche food markets, Myanmar seems to be on the cusp of transformation.

Richard Vines in *Bloomberg Business* elegantly depicts modern Myanmar: "It's happy hour in the bar of The Strand Hotel in Yangon. A smartly dressed barman mixes a Strand Sour as fans slowly revolve below the high ceiling. Musicians play. Tourists at tables beside the teak-lined walls check guidebooks and discuss where to go for dinner." He also describes an $87 tasting menu at a villa on Inya Lake featuring "lobster salad, veal fillet in pistachio crust, and Grand Marnier soufflé with orange sauce."

In addition to the flourishing food scene, the high-altitude Shan State is also participating in the "new latitude" wine phenomenon, highlighting grapes grown in the tropics, close to the equator. India, Indonesia, Cambodia, Vietnam, and Myanmar are among these producers where cool nights, limestone-based soils, modern viticulture techniques—and likely climate change—are to credit for their success. Breaking free from the approximately 30° to 50° latitude once considered suitable for quality wine production, a few vineyards in the Shan State are working tirelessly to invent a lasting wine culture in Myanmar.

Organic produce certification, production, and exportation are also on the rise. A local entrepreneur was the first to earn certification by an international organization in Myanmar. He described the honor: "It's a feather in the cap for the Ta'ang (Palaung) region, better known for fighting and opium cultivation." Although the initial goal of certification was to compete with the dominating Chinese tea imports, accreditation fortuitously created a new export niche, fermented green tea leaves.

CREATING A MODERN VERSION OF THE TEA LEAF SALAD: NO DIRT PIT (OR PASSPORT) REQUIRED

Myanmar used to be the only country where tea leaves were eaten. Demand in the West is on the rise due to the number of restaurants in the West owned by immigrants of Myanmar, coupled with how popular the tea leaf salad has become. Even so, getting your hands on the iconic leaves can be a challenge. It has been said that many restaurateurs make multiple trips to Myanmar each year, returning with suitcases full of the cured leaves. Others recruit small, local family producers to export the leaves specifically for them.

My goal was to create a modern version of fermented tea leaves that rival the authentic ones in flavor and, most important, can be replicated in the home kitchen, no dirt pit required. The San Francisco Bay Area is home to at least thirty Burmese restaurants, and tens of thousands of people in the local Burmese community. California's Burmese cuisine is so progressive that it tends to ride the line between authentic and New American, and allows creative freedom to merge cuisines in a modern way.

Once I began my research, I learned how sacred—and secretive, really—the method for fermenting tea leaves truly is. The chefs who create their fermented tea leaves in-house were generally not open to sharing their process. So, I ate. And ate. Sometimes in the dark corners of Burmese restaurants, alone, with my eyes closed to fully sense the nuanced flavors. Over the course of six months, I ate more tea leaf salads,

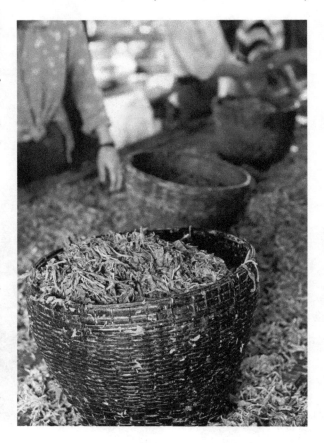

and fermented tea leaves by themselves, than is likely healthy for one human being. Still, the more I ate, the more I fell in love and found an interconnectedness with this powerful, vibrant dish.

Several visits to my favorite organic and fair trade tea provider in San Anselmo, California, Desta Epicures Guild, brought forth the idea to create two versions of fermented tea leaves: green and black. Although the idea was somewhat unconventional, I was reminded that there are generally two types of tea drinkers.

And I was insatiably curious to know how these two interpretations would taste. To my surprise, they were both great in very unique ways.

The green tea is more closely aligned with the traditional tea leaf salad and imparts the signature astringent, bright notes with hints of floral. The black tea brings forth malty, smoky flavors that are deep and a little mysterious. If you decide to ferment your own tea leaves, see the following page for some recommendations.

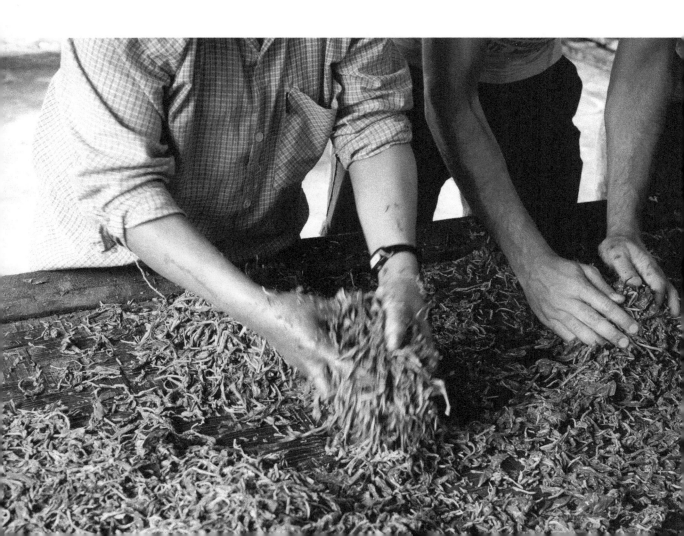

Fermented Tea Leaves, Two Ways

YIELD: ABOUT 3½ CUPS

2 cups organic whole dried green or black tea leaves

1½ cups roughly chopped Napa cabbage (about 1 small head)

2 medium shallots, roughly chopped

6 scallions, root end trimmed and roughly chopped

3-inch knob of ginger, peeled and roughly chopped

2 cloves garlic, roughly chopped

juice from 3 lemons

juice from 1 lime

¼ teaspoon dried chile pepper flakes

generous amount of sea salt

Here are a couple of tea recommendations to take you in the direction you choose to go:

GREEN TEA: *Dragonwell, one of China's most esteemed green teas, is pan-fried in large woks, often using bare hands. Like the first green vegetables in spring, it has a hint of sweetness, and a subtle roasted chestnut flavor that plays well off the dramatic citrus and ginger notes in the cured leaves.*

BLACK TEA: *Unlike green tea, black tea is oxidized by first heating and then rolling the leaves by hand or machine. This process causes the cell walls within the tea leaves to become damaged, releasing the oils. As a result, the leaves become darker and develop a more complex aroma and flavor. Two black teas seemed most approachable for this preparation:*

Darjeeling, also known as the champagne of teas, is grown at 1,600 feet in the Himalayan Mountains in India. Mildly astringent and with citrus and fruity notes of Muscat grape, Darjeeling rides the line between the typical flavor profiles found in black and green tea.

Assam is grown in northeastern India, one of the largest tea-growing regions in the world, bordering Bangladesh and Myanmar. This tea is grown at or near sea level and is known for its characteristic brisk, malty, and strong yet smooth flavor.

NOTE: *If possible, source an organic tea to avoid pesticides and other potential chemicals.*

Place the tea leaves in a medium bowl, and cover completely with hot water. Let soak for 10 to 15 minutes, until the leaves expand and soften. Drain and sort through the leaves for any stems or tough pieces. Squeeze the remaining liquid, and return the leaves to the same bowl, filled with lukewarm water this time. Smash the leaves with your hands to gently break them down. Repeat this process two more times. Next, fill the bowl with cold water, and let the leaves soak overnight to remove any remaining tannic and bitter notes.

The next morning, drain and place the tea leaves in a clean dish towel. Squeeze to remove the excess water, then place in a clean medium bowl.

In a food processor, combine the remaining ingredients, and pulse until a rough paste forms, scraping down the sides as you go. Add this mixture to the bowl with the tea leaves, and thoroughly combine with clean hands.

Transfer the mixture to two sterilized glass jars (1 pint and ½ pint). Fill the pint jar to the top, and place the remaining leaves in the ½ pint jar, pressing the mixture in both jars to remove any air bubbles. Cover both tightly, and store in a cool, dark pantry for 2 to 3 days to ferment, turning upside down a couple of times to evenly distribute the liquid. Then place the jars in the refrigerator until ready to use. The leaves will remain fresh in the refrigerator for up to a month.

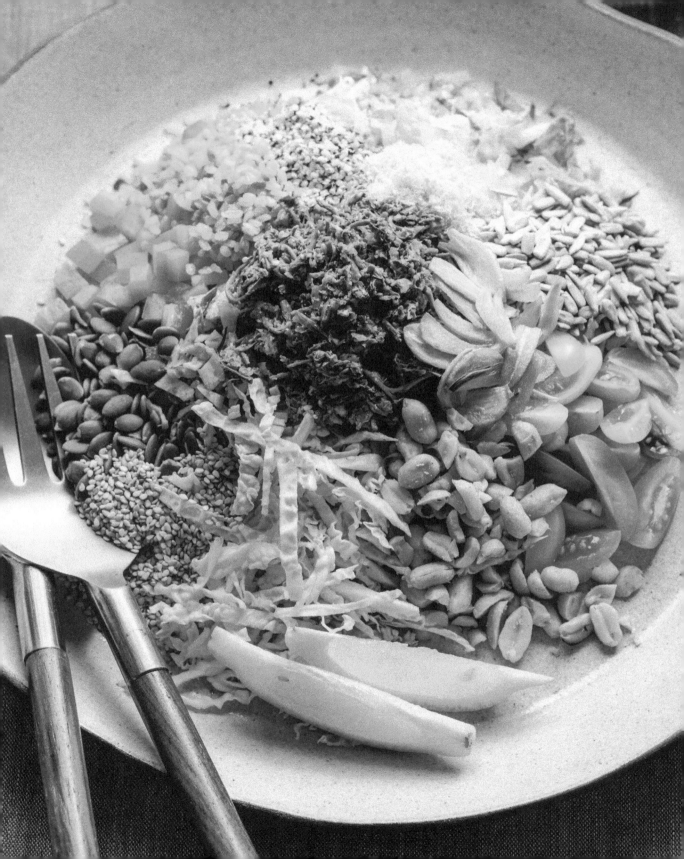

The Burmese Tea Leaf Salad

This salad has become a cult favorite for a very good reason: It's outrageously tasty, exhilarating to eat, and ignites all the senses. I'll admit it. I have a long-standing love affair with this salad. I often crave it, deeply. The variation of ingredients doesn't even matter that much. As long as it's made well, with perfectly bright, tart, and deeply flavored tea leaves, anything else pretty much goes. My modern version incorporates a few non-traditional ingredients, like romaine lettuce, red bell pepper, and a wide variety of seeds for added color, texture, and nutrients. Also, instead of fried beans or peas, I developed a recipe for roasted split mung dal. They're a slightly nutty, super healthy, and extra crunchy addition to an already exceptional lineup of ingredients.

NOTE: *Dried shrimp are widely used in Asian and Latin American kitchens. Their aroma is much stronger than their flavor, and they fade into the background while greatly enhancing whatever they come into contact with. Well-stocked Asian markets and large grocery stores often carry them. For a vegetarian version, omit the dried shrimp and fish sauce, and instead use tamari or soy sauce.*

Place the tea leaves in a fine-mesh sieve to allow any excess liquid to drain. Assemble the Napa cabbage, romaine, tomato, bell pepper, mung dal, seeds, peanuts, crispy garlic, and dried shrimp on a large platter or on individual plates. Add the desired amount of tea leaves, and drizzle the garlic oil and fish sauce over the salad.

At tableside, toss thoroughly with a spoon and fork or clean bare hands, until the tea leaves are completely incorporated with the other ingredients. Serve the lemon wedges on the side and Maldon sea salt for finishing.

SERVES 4

3 cups Fermented Tea Leaves (page 7)

4 cups finely shredded Napa cabbage (about 1 large head)

4 cups finely shredded romaine lettuce hearts (about 2 medium)

2 cups thinly sliced tomato

2 cups finely diced red bell pepper

½ cup Crunchy Roasted Split Mung Dal (page 86)

¼ cup raw, shelled, and unsalted sunflower seeds

¼ cup raw, unsalted pumpkin seeds

¼ cup raw sesame seeds, toasted

2 tablespoons raw hemp seeds

¼ cup, plus 2 tablespoons roughly chopped Roasted Peanuts (page 84)

½ cup Crispy Garlic (page 89), some slices left intact, others finely chopped

¼ cup finely ground dried shrimp

½ cup Garlic Oil (page 89)

2 teaspoons fish sauce

2 lemons, quartered

sea salt, plus Maldon sea salt for finishing

BALANCING FLAVORS

Each of us perceives taste differently, according to our DNA. Even more, we all possess different numbers of taste buds. Those with a greater number are often referred to as "supertasters." This group makes up about 25 percent of the population and has the ability to taste minor subtleties others can't. Individuals in this group may also have a strong dislike for certain foods, especially those with bitter characteristics, such as coffee and some cruciferous vegetables. On the opposite side of the spectrum are the "subtasters," who are less sensitive, and the "non-tasters," who have a small number of taste buds and characterize many foods as indistinctive. Everyone else falls under the category of "average taster."

Part art form, part science, balancing flavors is unique to each of us. The one common element is that each of the five tastes—salty, sweet, sour, bitter, and umami—must be represented individually and collectively for a dish to really shine. These five tastes are common in the West. Burmese cuisine also applies a sixth taste, astringent, as described below. The tea leaf salad, and many other Burmese salads, are excellent examples of this diversity and balance of flavor. Beyond creating outrageously delicious food by bringing flavors into balance, incorporating the full spectrum of tastes also brings forth a vital symmetry in mind-body physiology. In other words, when each of these tastes is represented in a dish, most, if not all, nutrients are available, and a state of authentic satisfaction can be achieved.

As you cook, taste often. Think of the multiple flavors, and bring your intuition to the game. The win is found by learning to riff on a recipe, altering it based on your palate and the ingredients in your kitchen, and accomplishing a sense of "roundness"—that unmistakable balance when the ingredients speak for themselves and align in a harmonious way.

The recipes in this book are intended to serve as inspiration, loose guides. My hope is that you'll listen to your intuition in the kitchen and make them your own. To effectively manipulate and enhance the flavors to suit your individual palate, here's a quick guide on balancing flavors.

SALTY: Salt not only enhances the appetite, but it also pulls sweet notes forward while suppressing bitter characteristics. If a dish just needs "something" or is too bitter, try salt first. And go sparingly. It's easy to add, but not as easy to deduct. If you go too far, dilute with a little water. Adding a touch of sweetener may also do the trick to bring the salt back into balance.

SWEET: Of all the tastes, sweet has the greatest soothing effect on the body and is also required in the largest amount to be detected by the taste buds. It complements sour, bitter, and salty notes best. In small quantities, it delivers an undeniable completeness to savory food. If something is too bitter or too sour, try adding more sweetener. If the sweet note becomes too intense, add something sour such as vinegar or lemon.

SOUR: Often referred to as acid, this element provides that irresistible brightness, that coveted high note. Sour is second in line of importance, next to salt, for balancing savory food. Citrus and vinegar are two of the most commonly used sour ingredients, and vinaigrettes are excellent for providing this component to a dish. Just keep in mind that balancing acidity with the other tastes is vital to the outcome of the finished dish. If you taste a dish and it falls flat, try adding a little salt first. If it still needs "something," add extra lemon or vinegar, whatever works best with the other ingredients. And if you happen to take it too far, add a little sweetener to bring everything back into balance.

BITTER: Of all the tastes, the human palate is the most sensitive to bitter notes in food, likely due to the fact that many bitter substances found in nature are toxic. Bitter flavors assist in the detoxification process and fat metabolism, and are vital to overall health. Add more bitter ingredients, such as grapefruit or leafy greens, if the dish is too rich or too sweet. To cut bitter notes, add a little salt first, then try a sweetener if the dish needs more roundness.

UMAMI: This strong and savory flavor is not easy to resist. Mushrooms, fermented foods, some cheeses, fish sauce, slow-cooked meats, and nutritional yeast provide those deep flavors (the low notes) to food. When a dish seems balanced otherwise, but could use more depth, try adding a umami ingredient. Just be aware that too much can completely dismantle the other flavors. If this happens, add more of the other flavors to bring the dish back into harmony.

ASTRINGENT: Often derived from ingredients such as green tea, the astringent flavor comes across as dry, like the fuzzy feeling left on the tongue after drinking red wine, or green or black tea. Some say it's not even a taste but rather a tactile sensation. The benefit is that it provides the sought-after balance, structure, and complexity often celebrated in Burmese cuisine. Astringency can balance excessive sweetness and vice versa. Other foods that deliver the astringent quality include lentils, beans, pomegranate, green apple, pear, sprouts, and cauliflower.

THE INSPIRATION

When I first started writing this book and began sharing the concept with friends, some people responded with a look of bewilderment. Every time, that reaction gave me pause. Not because I didn't love the story, but I started to wonder how I was going to honor the richness and meaning behind the iconic tea leaf salad, especially to those who haven't been fortunate enough to taste it. Even more, how was I going to translate that depth and gravity throughout the other recipes? This is a salad unlike any other.

When I moved toward this uncertainty instead of resisting it, I was able to connect with the reasons this salad is so alluring: It is full of fascinating, contradictory flavors and textures. Within those connected moments, floods of inspiration came my way. At times, it was overwhelming. Author Amy Tan dug deep in her playful TED Talk, *Where Does Creativity Hide?*, describing these moments as "the arrival of luck." And while I felt fortunate, harnessing that energy, that luck, was often a challenge. Then I decided I didn't have to. Actually, that I couldn't.

So I set off on an expedition of whimsical curiosity, chasing the innovative, the unidentified, in pursuit of those contradictions: tart and sweet; salty and bitter; crunchy and tender; spicy and cool; fresh and cooked. Combined, these elements make the tea leaf salad complete. That balance, those surprising details, were vital to replicate throughout the remainder of the recipes.

Within these pages you'll find the following combinations: green mango with tangles of slippery noodles, vibrant citrus, and deep-ruby-red chile oil; smoky, spicy kimchi with sweet star anise and maple pork; saffron, tart green apple, and garlic prawns; bright preserved lemon, creamy goat cheese, and tart sumac; sweet watermelon, farro, grilled halloumi, and floral pink peppercorn; and briny sea scallops with crushed chamomile-grapefruit salt.

There's also a pantry section with infused oils, spice blends, crunchy legumes, toasted chickpea flour, and time-honored methods such as fermentation and pickling, all of which provide even greater depth and make this food especially vibrant. To get the most out of these recipes, I recommend browsing through the pantry section before you begin cooking. Many of the recipes incorporate these essential items, and some require advanced preparation.

These dynamic dishes are intended to be presented in a deconstructed format (or tossed tableside) similar to the tea leaf salad. They are meant to be shared. When we're able to sit down and mindfully connect, understand, and respect one another through food, conflict of ideologies often can be set aside. Only then are we able to remember our shared basic humanity. And when the focal point is fresh, intense food, an elevated interaction is likely.

The tea leaf salad commands that interaction and presence. Listen to what happens with your first bite: bold crunching and slight pops. See the rich, multidimensional colors and textures. Smell the fresh garlic, citrus, ginger, and chiles. Feel the firm, silky, rough, and smooth elements. Simply allow the ingredients to speak for themselves.

Innately, from these harmonious contradictions and diverse ingredients comes health. These salads are deeply flavorful, and they are also intended to optimize well-being. I believe that food is information for the body. And the people of Myanmar instinctively know that, for example, a pinch of turmeric not only elevates flavor but is a powerful anti-inflammatory, so critical for the prevention of most major diseases.

These same components, to elevate well-being and vitality, are weaved throughout the recipes. For instance, Golden Vinaigrette (page 61) is deeply infused with fresh carrot juice, healthy fats for nutrient absorption, and copious amounts of ground turmeric. And Coconut-Matcha Jeweled Rice Salad (page 44) is slowly simmered with creamy coconut milk and matcha, a premium ground green tea with remarkable antioxidant benefits, including the powerful polyphenol, EGCG.

We currently live in the golden age of wellness. Awareness about the connection between eating whole, nutrient-dense food and leading a happy, balanced life is heightened. Fresh organic food, made from scratch, has the potential to make us feel invigorated and alive. This belief is the crux of the book.

The final core element to this story is honoring the sense of adventure found through food. Now more than ever, there is a deep longing to experience the world. Merging culinary traditions allows us to sit at the fringe of multiple cultures. There, we can be quickly transported and view the world through a different lens. Food is at the heart of a culture, after all. With Myanmar and Southeast Asian cuisine as my touchstones, I found the process of incorporating New American and international concepts throughout the remaining recipes thrilling. There's an undeniable distortion when various cuisines collide. The true beauty is found when the flavors realign and a new form of order returns.

As the resilient people of Myanmar have so brilliantly illustrated for centuries, there's an elemental connection between food and love: a source of kinship and sanctuary discovered through those simple rhythms of living. There's an opportunity for renewal by nourishing ourselves with food that surprises, that makes us feel alive. The vibrancy of fresh ingredients, recipes steeped in tradition and meaning, and the intentional sharing of meals—this is the definition of power itself. I believe so many of our modern hardships could be solved if we simply decided to take a seat at each other's table more often.

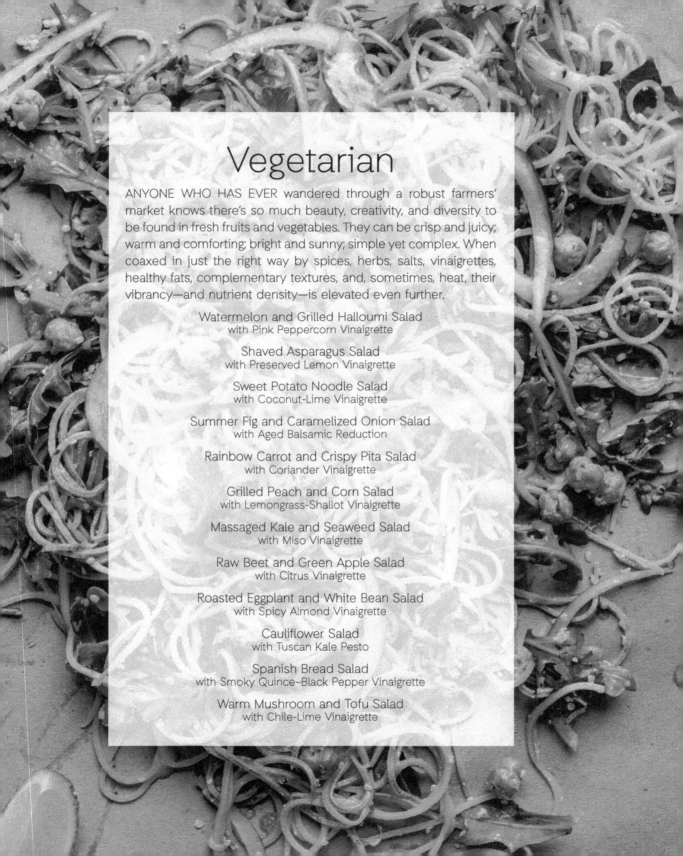

Vegetarian

ANYONE WHO HAS EVER wandered through a robust farmers' market knows there's so much beauty, creativity, and diversity to be found in fresh fruits and vegetables. They can be crisp and juicy; warm and comforting; bright and sunny; simple yet complex. When coaxed in just the right way by spices, herbs, salts, vinaigrettes, healthy fats, complementary textures, and, sometimes, heat, their vibrancy—and nutrient density—is elevated even further.

Watermelon and Grilled Halloumi Salad
with Pink Peppercorn Vinaigrette

Shaved Asparagus Salad
with Preserved Lemon Vinaigrette

Sweet Potato Noodle Salad
with Coconut-Lime Vinaigrette

Summer Fig and Caramelized Onion Salad
with Aged Balsamic Reduction

Rainbow Carrot and Crispy Pita Salad
with Coriander Vinaigrette

Grilled Peach and Corn Salad
with Lemongrass-Shallot Vinaigrette

Massaged Kale and Seaweed Salad
with Miso Vinaigrette

Raw Beet and Green Apple Salad
with Citrus Vinaigrette

Roasted Eggplant and White Bean Salad
with Spicy Almond Vinaigrette

Cauliflower Salad
with Tuscan Kale Pesto

Spanish Bread Salad
with Smoky Quince–Black Pepper Vinaigrette

Warm Mushroom and Tofu Salad
with Chile-Lime Vinaigrette

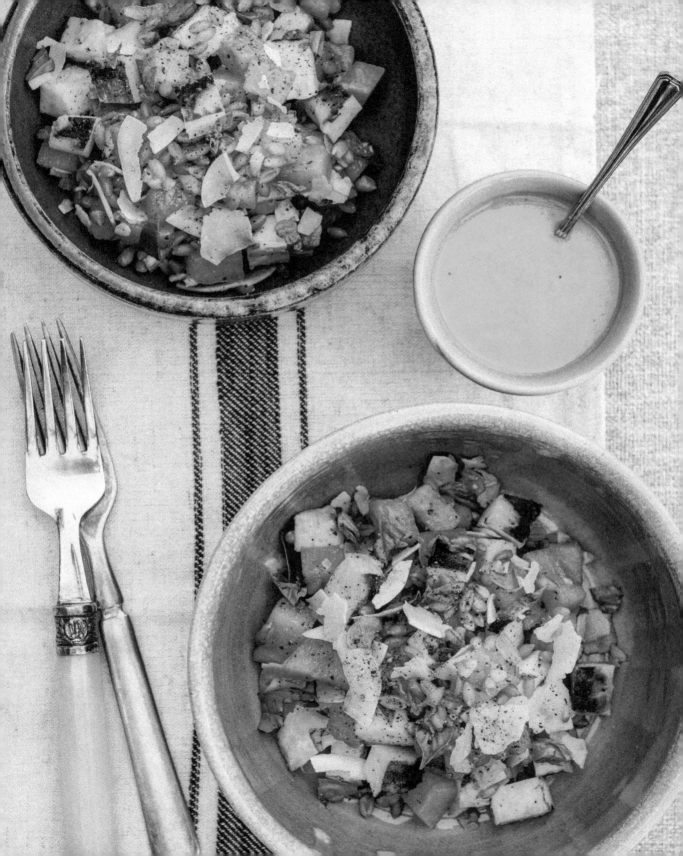

Watermelon and Grilled Halloumi Salad
with Pink Peppercorn Vinaigrette

In the heat of summer, it's no wonder why watermelon graces almost every table. It is refreshingly sweet and intoxicatingly juicy. In this dish, the ultra-salty grilled halloumi cheese, made from a combination of goat and sheep's milk and originating from Cyprus, and floral notes from the pink peppercorns temper the sweetness while still allowing the star ingredient, watermelon, to shine.

SERVES 4

1 medium watermelon (about 3–4 pounds), divided

1½ teaspoons whole pink peppercorns, finely ground

2 tablespoons champagne vinegar

juice of 1 lime

1½ teaspoons red chile flakes, divided

1 clove garlic

¼ cup, plus 1 tablespoon grapeseed oil, divided

8 ounces halloumi cheese, sliced in half lengthwise

2 cups cooked and cooled farro

¼ cup roughly torn fresh basil

¼ cup unsweetened coconut flakes

sea salt and freshly cracked black pepper

Slice the watermelon in half. Reserve about a quarter of the melon for the vinaigrette, and slice the remainder into ½-inch cubes until you have about 2½ to 3 cups. Set aside.

For the vinaigrette, add about 1 cup of roughly chopped watermelon along with the ground pink peppercorns, vinegar, lime juice, ½ teaspoon of the chile flakes, and garlic to a blender, and pulse until smooth. With the motor running, drizzle in ¼ cup of the grapeseed oil until emulsified, and season with salt and pepper. Transfer to a glass jar, and refrigerate until ready to use. It's perfectly normal for this vinaigrette to separate. Shake well before assembling the salad.

Next, drizzle the remaining 1 tablespoon of grapeseed oil over the halloumi cheese. Preheat your grill to medium-high (an indoor grill pan or heavy skillet may be used instead). Grill each piece of cheese for about 1 minute per side, or until light grill marks form. Remove from the heat, and allow to cool slightly. Slice into ¼-inch cubes, and set aside.

To assemble the salad, arrange the cubed watermelon, farro, and cheese on a large serving platter or on individual plates. Scatter the basil, coconut flakes, the remaining 1 teaspoon of chile flakes, and, if desired, extra black pepper over the top. Serve with the vinaigrette on the side.

Shaved Asparagus Salad
with Preserved Lemon Vinaigrette

SERVES 4

2 tablespoons finely diced Preserved Lemon (page 85), white pith removed, or 1½ tablespoons fresh lemon zest

juice from 2 lemons

1 teaspoon maple syrup, grade B

1 cup extra virgin olive oil

2 pounds asparagus, ends trimmed

2 cups pea shoots

½ pound goat cheese, crumbled

1 cup roughly chopped pistachios, with some large pieces and some "dust"

sea salt and freshly cracked black pepper, plus Maldon sea salt for finishing

I tend to like things uncomplicated: my kitchen pantry, my relationships, and my daily schedule. We all know life doesn't always ebb in that direction. And when it doesn't, it's comforting to know we have some command over the little things, like what we eat. This salad hits many high notes with tangy preserved lemon vinaigrette and creamy goat cheese. However, as a whole, it's so simple and effortless.

For the vinaigrette, combine the preserved lemon or lemon zest, lemon juice, maple syrup, sea salt, and pepper in a bowl. Slowly whisk in the olive oil until emulsified. Transfer the vinaigrette to a glass jar. Use immediately or refrigerate for up to a week. Shake before using as the preserved lemon or lemon zest will likely settle to the bottom.

Next, in a large bowl, add ¼ cup plus 2 tablespoons of the vinaigrette. Using a vegetable peeler, shave the asparagus into long ribbons. If the stalk becomes difficult to shave as it gets smaller, grab a wooden spoon and hold the stalk on top of the handle. This should give you some leverage to effectively shave the remainder. Leave the tips intact, if possible.

Transfer the asparagus to the bowl with the vinaigrette, and gently toss to coat. Let sit for 5 to 10 minutes to soften somewhat. Toss the pea shoots with another 2 tablespoons of the vinaigrette. Season both the asparagus and pea shoots with salt and pepper right before assembling the salad.

Arrange the shaved asparagus, pea shoots, goat cheese, and pistachios on a large platter or on individual plates. Serve with extra vinaigrette, Maldon sea salt, and pepper on the side.

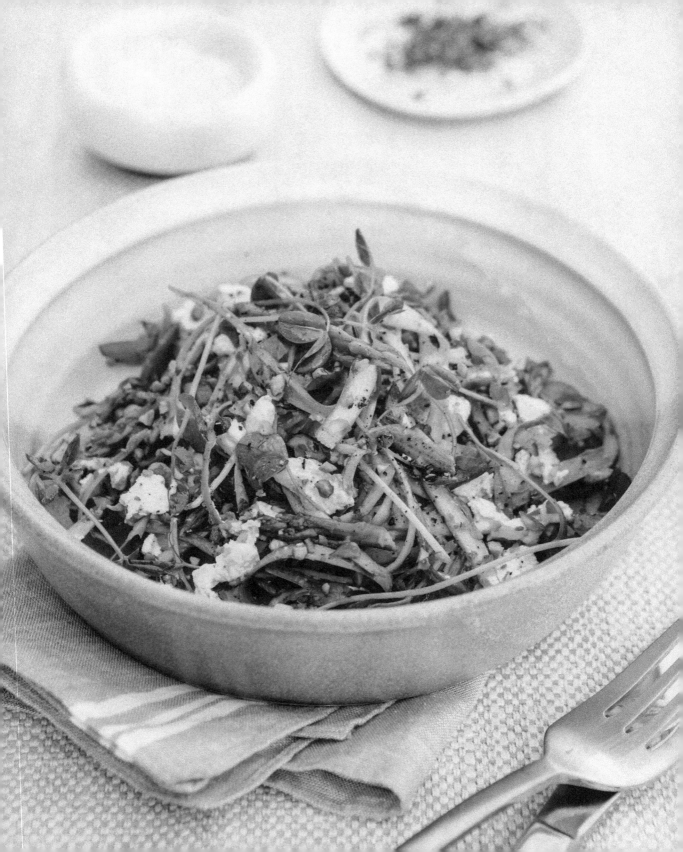

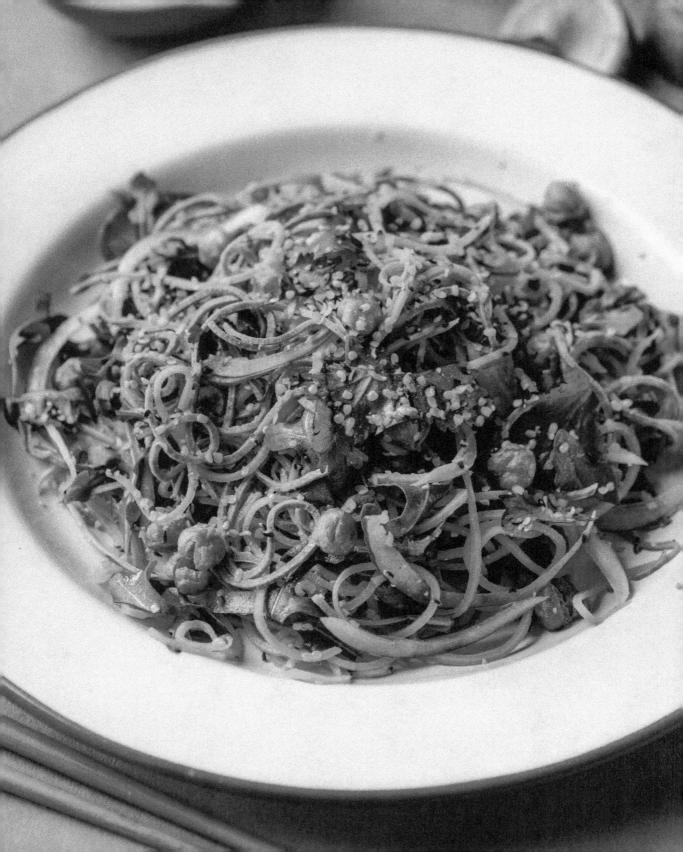

Sweet Potato Noodle Salad
with Coconut-Lime Vinaigrette

I'm of the opinion that an entire cookbook could be dedicated solely to sweet potatoes, a rich source of antioxidants and anti-inflammatory nutrients. Some countries, such as India and Uganda, rely on this year-round root vegetable to provide children with sufficient vitamin A. Studies also reveal sweet potatoes may have more bioavailable beta-carotene than dark green, leafy vegetables. These noodles are lightly blanched, and paired with the health-promoting fat found in coconut, allowing the body to assimilate the benefits in a creamy, tangy, crunchy way.

To make the vinaigrette, combine the coconut milk, lime juice, and garlic. Slowly whisk in ¾ cup of the grapeseed oil until emulsified. Season with salt and pepper, and transfer to a glass jar. Store in the refrigerator for up to a week.

Preheat the oven to 400°F, and line a baking sheet with parchment. Toss the chickpeas with the remaining 2 tablespoons of grapeseed oil and the cumin. Season with salt and pepper, and bake for 45 to 50 minutes, tossing once halfway through baking. When done, the beans should be golden brown and crunchy. Once cooled, they will crisp even further.

To make the noodles, use a spiralizer with a 1.2 x 2 mm blade, or a vegetable peeler if you don't have a spiralizer. A lot of the nutrition is in the skin of the sweet potato, so I like to leave it on. Peeling the sweet potatoes first is also an option, however. Bring a large pot of water to a boil, turn off the heat, and blanch the noodles for about 4 to 5 minutes, or until they begin to soften. Drain and rinse with cold water to stop the cooking process. Shake off the excess water before assembling the salad.

Toss the noodles, beans, arugula, drained red onion slices, and cilantro in a large serving bowl with the desired amount of vinaigrette. Garnish with hemp seeds, chile flakes, and additional chopped cilantro. Season with Maldon sea salt and black pepper.

SERVES 4

1 cup coconut milk

juice of 4 limes

2 cloves garlic, finely diced

¾ cup, plus 2 tablespoons grapeseed oil, divided

2 cups cooked chickpeas

1 tablespoon ground cumin

2–3 large sweet potatoes (about 8 cups of "noodles")

4 cups roughly chopped arugula

1 cup very thinly sliced red onion, soaked in cold water for 15 minutes

1 cup roughly chopped cilantro, plus extra for garnish

¼ cup raw hemp seeds

1 tablespoon dried chile pepper flakes

sea salt and freshly cracked black pepper, plus Maldon sea salt to finish

Summer Fig and Caramelized Onion Salad
with Aged Balsamic Reduction

SERVES 4

1 cup aged balsamic vinegar (preferably at least 12 years)

½ teaspoon Herbes de Provence

1 clove garlic, finely diced

2 tablespoons extra virgin olive oil, divided

1 tablespoon grapeseed oil

1 large yellow onion, quartered and thinly sliced

2 cups thinly shaved fresh fennel, placed in ice water until ready to assemble

2 pints mixed fresh figs (about 2 pounds), sliced into various sizes

4 cups packed spinach, thinly sliced into strips

¾ cup walnuts, toasted and then roughly chopped

½ pound blue cheese, broken into bite-size pieces

¼ cup microgreens (optional)

sea salt and freshly cracked black pepper, plus Maldon sea salt for finishing

For years, this has been my go-to flavor combination for parties because of its broad appeal and versatility. California figs are available almost year-round, but the richest, most decadent fruit typically hits in August through early October. It's worth seeking out a couple of varieties for this salad. And if blue cheese isn't your thing, an earthy triple crème brie can easily stand in.

For the balsamic reduction, combine the balsamic vinegar, Herbes de Provence, and garlic in a medium saucepan. Bring the mixture to a boil over medium-high heat, then turn off the heat, allowing the garlic to lightly infuse the vinegar. Season with salt and pepper. Once cool, slowly whisk in 1 tablespoon of the olive oil until combined. Use immediately, or store in a glass jar in the refrigerator for up to a week. Bring the balsamic reduction to room temperature before using it because it becomes very thick when cold.

Next, caramelize the onion. Add the grapeseed oil and onion to a medium sauté pan over medium-high heat. Once the onion just begins to turn a light golden color, reduce the heat to low. Allow to cook for 30 to 40 minutes, stirring frequently, until the onion becomes very soft and a deep caramel color develops. To prevent sticking, feel free to add a small amount of water. Remove from the heat, and allow to cool. Then transfer to an airtight container, and store in the refrigerator for up to 5 days.

To assemble the salad, drain the fennel and dry well. Toss the spinach and fennel with the remaining 1 tablespoon of olive oil, and season with salt and pepper. Arrange the figs, fennel, spinach, caramelized onion, walnuts, and cheese on a large platter or on individual plates. Sprinkle with Maldon sea salt and black pepper, if desired. Garnish with microgreens, if using, and serve the balsamic reduction on the side.

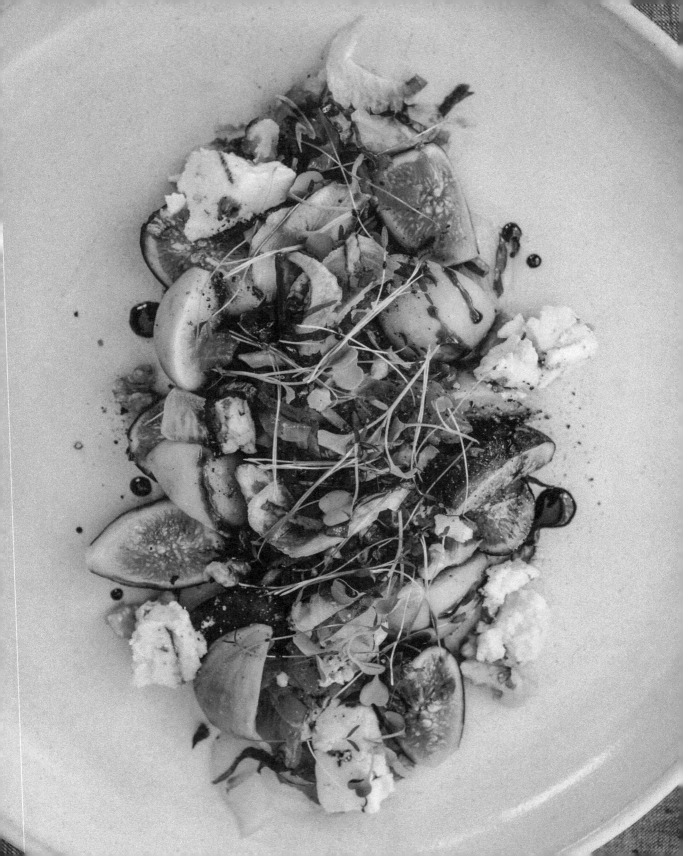

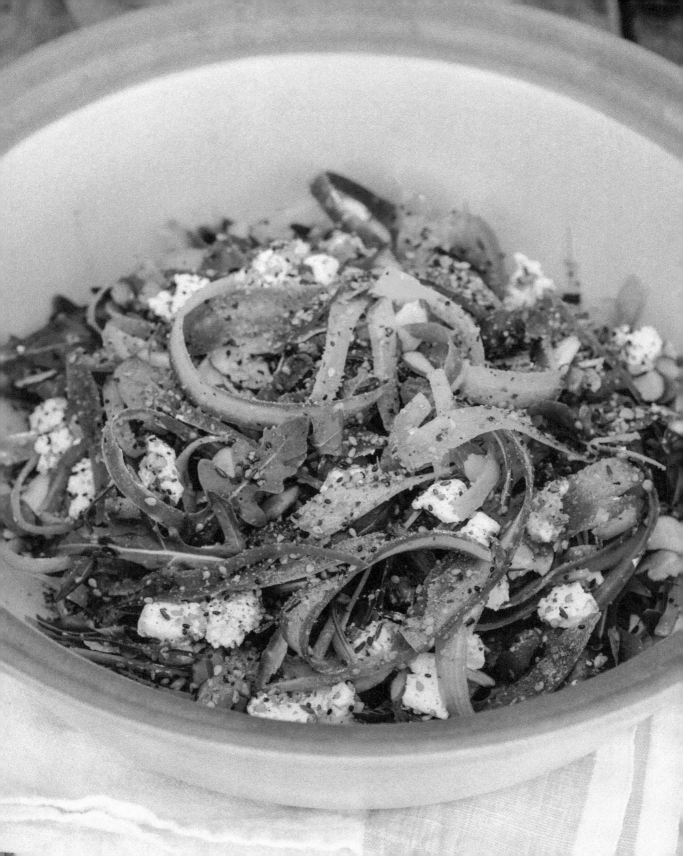

Rainbow Carrot and Crispy Pita Salad
with Coriander Vinaigrette

The vibrant colors and textures of this lively salad quickly transport you to the Middle East. The distinct ingredient is the Egyptian seed, nut, and spice blend called dukkah (pronounced DOO-kah). Derived from the Arabic word dakka, *which means "to crush," it is a highly versatile and nutrient-dense condiment. For the olives, bright-green Sicilian Castelvetrano is a good choice.*

Combine the ground coriander, preserved lemon or lemon zest, shallot, diced garlic, vinegar, and maple syrup in a medium bowl. Slowly whisk in ¾ cup of the olive oil, and season with salt and pepper. Transfer the vinaigrette to a glass jar, and refrigerate for up to a week. Shake before using as the preserved lemon or lemon zest will likely settle to the bottom.

Preheat the oven to 375°F. Separate each pita into two thin rounds by cutting along the edge and gently pulling apart. In a small bowl, combine the remaining 2 tablespoons of olive oil with the sumac, salt, and pepper. Rub each pita half generously with the sliced garlic, then tear the pita into jagged pieces. Place on two parchment-lined baking sheets, and brush each piece with the olive oil mixture. Bake for 10 to 12 minutes, or until the pita pieces begin to turn golden and crisp on the edges. Remove, and allow to cool before serving. Any extra can be stored in an airtight container for up to a week.

Toss the carrots with a tablespoon or two of the vinaigrette in a large bowl, and season with salt and pepper. Allow to sit for 10 minutes to soften slightly. Add the arugula, almonds, raisins, olives, goat cheese, and mint to the carrots, and toss with additional vinaigrette. Serve on individual plates and garnish with extra mint leaves and dukkah. Serve the pita crisps on the side.

SERVES 4

2 tablespoons whole coriander, toasted and finely ground

2 tablespoons Preserved Lemon (page 85) or 1 tablespoon fresh lemon zest

2 tablespoons finely diced shallot

4 cloves garlic, 2 finely diced and 2 sliced in half

¼ cup, plus 2 tablespoons champagne vinegar

1 teaspoon maple syrup, grade B

¾ cup, plus 2 tablespoons extra virgin olive oil, divided

2 (6–8-inch) whole grain pitas

1 teaspoon salt-free ground sumac

8 large rainbow carrots, peeled and shaved into ribbons with a vegetable peeler

4 cups arugula or other peppery green

½ cup slivered almonds

½ cup golden raisins

½ cup green olives, pitted and roughly chopped

4–6 ounces goat cheese

¼ cup roughly torn fresh mint leaves, plus extra for garnish

½ cup Dukkah (page 85)

sea salt and freshly cracked black pepper

Grilled Peach and Corn Salad
with Lemongrass-Shallot Vinaigrette

SERVES 4

1½ tablespoons finely grated lemongrass

3 tablespoons finely diced shallot

3 tablespoons umeboshi plum vinegar (or red wine vinegar)

1 tablespoon maple syrup, grade B

1 cup, plus 3 tablespoons grapeseed oil, divided

2–3 large peaches, sliced in half, pits removed

4 ears of corn, shucked and silks removed

4 cups arugula

1 cup roughly torn radicchio

¼ cup thinly sliced jalapeño, seeds and ribs removed

¼ cup toasted and roughly chopped pistachios

¼ cup toasted sesame seeds

2 tablespoons finely diced Pickled Ginger (page 87)

sea salt and freshly cracked black pepper, plus Maldon sea salt for finishing

In the heat of summer, when stone fruit is at its peak, grilled peaches are my favorite ingredient in everything from savory to sweet preparations. This salad, with its complex contradictory and bright complementary flavors, is full of lively surprises.

NOTE: *Umeboshi plum vinegar is the by-product of the Japanese umeboshi-making process. When preserved with shiso leaves, the result is a vibrant pinkish-red, sour and salty condiment.*

For the vinaigrette, whisk together the lemongrass, shallot, vinegar, and maple syrup in a medium bowl. Slowly whisk in 1 cup, plus 2 tablespoons of the grapeseed oil. If using umeboshi plum vinegar, you probably won't need to add salt at this point. Otherwise, season to taste. Transfer to a glass jar, and refrigerate for up to 5 days. Shake before assembling the salad as the vinaigrette will likely separate.

Next, preheat the grill, indoor grill pan, or heavy skillet to medium-high. Coat the peaches and corn with the remaining 1 tablespoon of grapeseed oil, and season with salt and pepper. Grill the peaches for 1 to 2 minutes per side, or until grill marks form and the fruit begins to soften and caramelize. The corn may take slightly longer, about 5 to 6 minutes. Remove both from the heat, and allow to cool. Once cool, gently slice the peaches into bite-size pieces. With a sharp knife, slice off the corn from each ear. Doing this in a large bowl makes for easier cleanup.

To assemble the salad, arrange the peaches, corn, arugula, radicchio, jalapeño, pistachios, sesame seeds, and pickled ginger on a large platter or on individual plates. Serve with the vinaigrette on the side, along with some Maldon sea salt and black pepper, if desired.

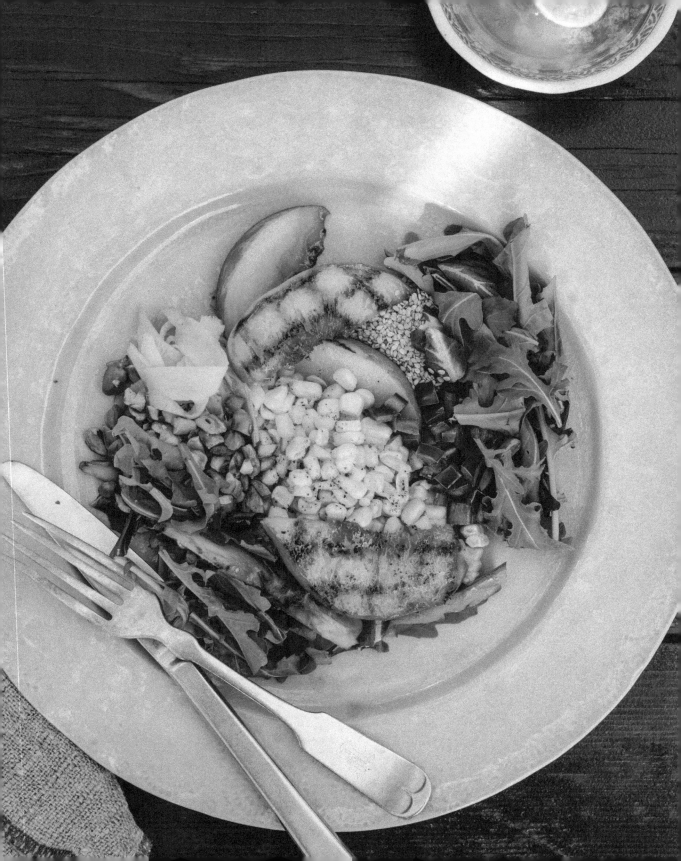

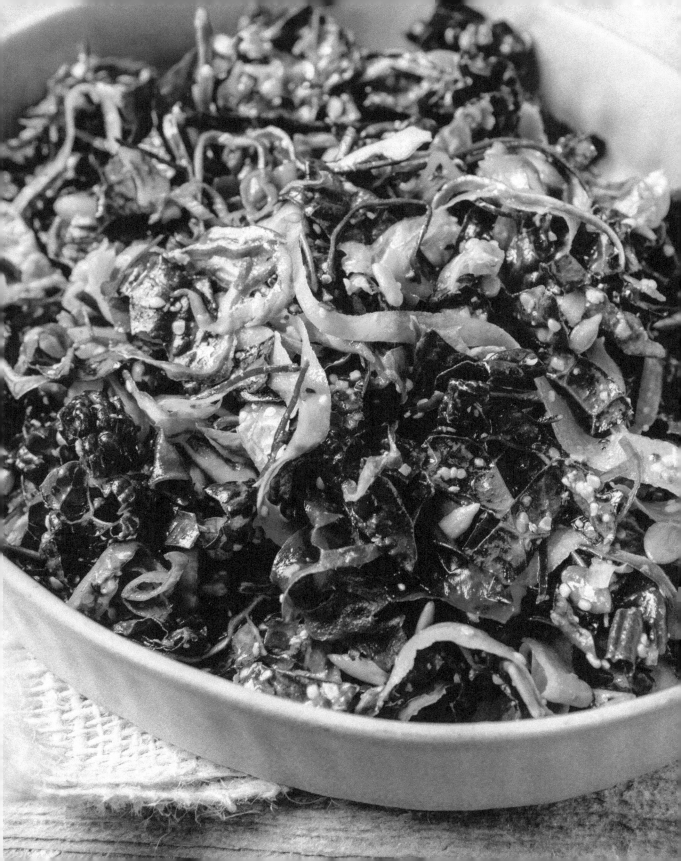

Massaged Kale and Seaweed Salad
with Miso Vinaigrette

This recipe transforms an otherwise sturdy green into something luscious by giving it a little friction, some salt, and a few minutes to hang out in the garlic-studded miso vinaigrette. The seed mixture provides crunch and texture, and creates a salad that is as nutrient dense as it is delicious.

NOTE: For thousands of years, Asian diets have relied on seaweed for its rich store of iodine, essential vitamins, and minerals. With well over thirty edible varieties of seaweed, mild arame is an approachable choice if you're new to the sea vegetable scene. Other choices include wakame, dulse, and hijiki, and incorporating a couple of varieties makes for an interesting salad.

SERVES 2–4

¼ cup white miso paste

1–2 cloves garlic, smashed into a paste

2 teaspoons umeboshi plum vinegar

2 tablespoons unseasoned rice vinegar

1 tablespoon fresh lemon juice

½ cup filtered water

¼ cup, plus 1 tablespoon extra virgin olive oil

2 medium bunches Tuscan kale, stems removed

3 medium heads romaine hearts

4 large carrots, peeled and shaved into thin ribbons with a vegetable peeler

4 cups seaweed, soaked in filtered water for 15 minutes or until soft, then drained thoroughly

4 cups finely shredded purple cabbage (about 1 medium head)

1 cup raw pumpkin seeds, plus extra for garnish

1 cup raw, shelled sunflower seeds, plus extra for garnish

1 cup raw hemp seeds, plus extra for garnish

½ cup finely chopped on the bias scallions

sea salt and freshly cracked black pepper

In a medium bowl, whisk together the miso paste, garlic, both vinegars, lemon juice, and filtered water until smooth. Slowly stream in the olive oil until emulsified. Season with salt and pepper, if needed. Transfer the vinaigrette to a glass jar, and refrigerate for up to 5 days.

To prepare the kale, stack 5 to 8 leaves on top of each other. Roll tightly into a log, and slice into a ⅛-inch chiffonade. Continue with the remaining kale. In a large bowl, add about ¼ cup of the vinaigrette. Place the kale on top, and lightly season with sea salt. With clean hands, gently massage the vinaigrette and salt into the kale until it begins to soften, adding more vinaigrette if necessary. At this point, you can either refrigerate the kale for up to 30 minutes or continue to assemble the salad. To chiffonade the romaine hearts, stack 4 to 5 leaves and slice them into ⅛-inch strips. Continue with the remaining romaine then add them to the kale mixture.

To assemble, add the carrot, seaweed, cabbage, seeds, and scallions to the kale mixture in a large bowl. Toss with additional vinaigrette, and taste, adding more salt and/or pepper, if necessary. Serve on individual plates and garnish with additional seeds, if desired.

Raw Beet and Green Apple Salad
with Citrus Vinaigrette

SERVES 4

¼ cup orange marmalade

1½ teaspoons Dijon mustard

½ cup apple cider vinegar

¼ cup, plus 2 tablespoons extra virgin olive oil

4 large beets, peeled, and finely shaved with a vegetable peeler (about 4–5 cups)

2 cups tangerine or orange segments

¾ cup toasted and roughly chopped walnuts

2 cups julienned green apples

¼ pound ricotta salata cheese, finely shaved with a vegetable peeler

¼ cup, plus 2 tablespoons whole fresh tarragon leaves

sea salt and freshly cracked black pepper, plus Maldon sea salt for finishing

As a child, many of my hours were spent at the kitchen table, long after the dishes had been cleared and the food put away. I would sit with a pile of canned beets on my plate, as they glared at me, in a heckling sort of way. They were disturbingly mushy with a strong metallic taste, and nothing good came of them. Thankfully, my first experience with fresh beets was an epiphany. Try the brilliant fuchsia and white-striped Italian Chioggia (kee-OH-jah) beets, if you can find them; their presentation is stunning. For the marmalade, I recommend Dundee brand, which uses Seville oranges from Scotland.

To make this simple citrus vinaigrette, whisk together the marmalade or jam, mustard, and vinegar in a medium bowl. Season with salt and pepper, and slowly stream in the olive oil until emulsified. Transfer to a glass jar and refrigerate for up to a week.

Place the shaved beets in a large bowl of ice water to retain their crispness while you prepare the other ingredients. Once ready to assemble the salad, drain and thoroughly dry the beets so the vinaigrette will adhere to them well.

To assemble the salad, toss the beets, tangerine or orange segments, walnuts, apple, and ricotta salata in a large bowl with the desired amount of vinaigrette. Serve on individual plates, garnish with tarragon leaves, and season with Maldon sea salt and pepper.

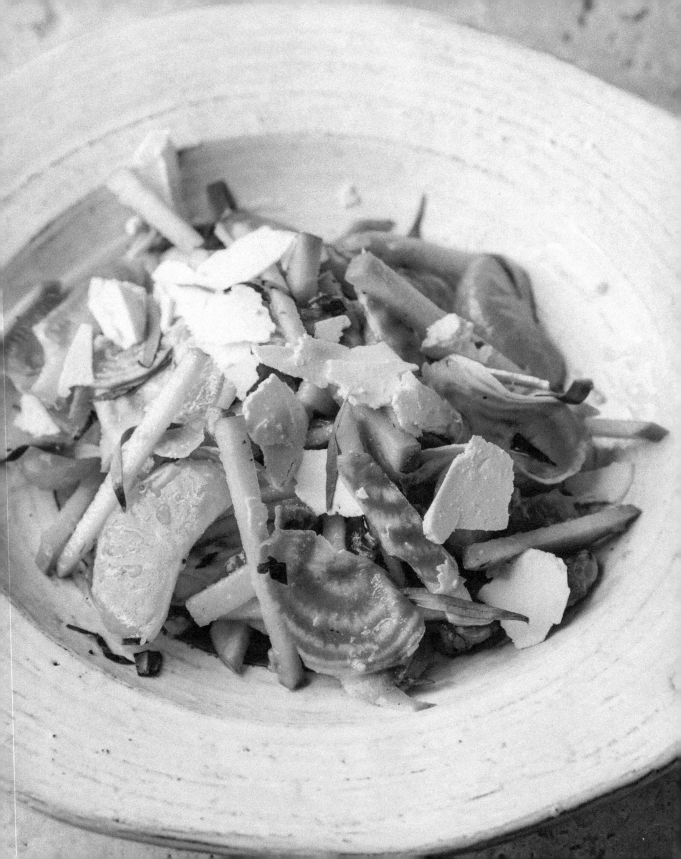

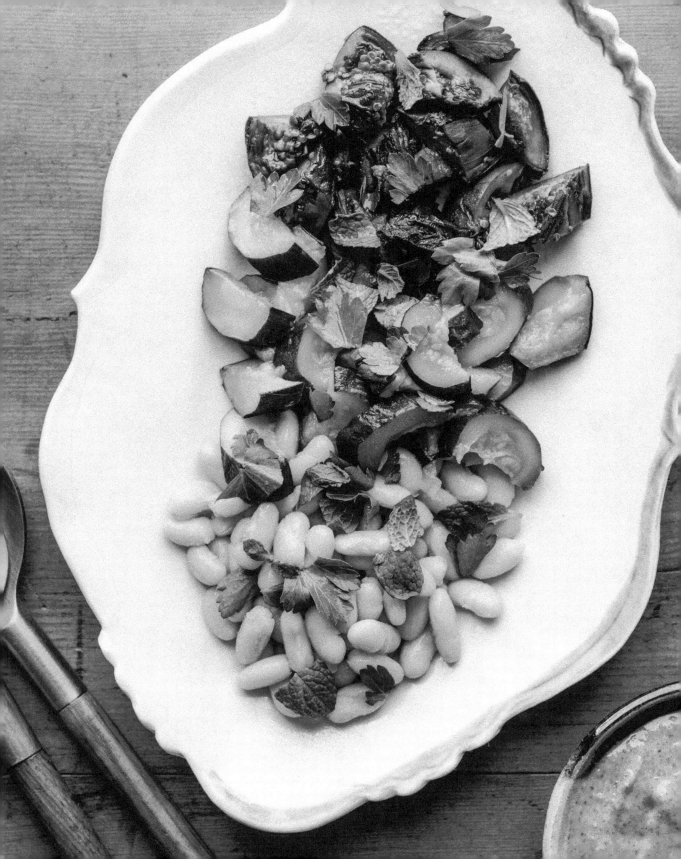

Roasted Eggplant and White Bean Salad
with Spicy Almond Vinaigrette

This vinaigrette is conceptualized around traditional peanut sauce widely used in the cuisines of Thailand, Vietnam, China, Indonesia, and sometimes sub-Saharan Africa. To mix things up, this recipe incorporates almonds blended with fiery red curry and earthy miso paste. The end result is deeply flavorful and oh so versatile.

SERVES 4

2 tablespoons white miso paste

¼ cup, plus 2 tablespoons almond butter

2 tablespoons red curry paste

2 tablespoons tamari or soy sauce

2 tablespoons mirin, or unseasoned rice vinegar with 1 teaspoon maple syrup added

¼ cup unseasoned rice vinegar

1 teaspoon dried chile pepper flakes

1–2 cloves garlic, finely diced

½ cup very warm water

3 medium eggplants (Listada work well) or 6 Japanese eggplants, sliced into quarters

4 medium zucchini, sliced in half lengthwise

3 tablespoons grapeseed oil, divided

3 cups cooked cannellini, navy, or other white beans

¼ cup roughly torn fresh mint

¼ cup roughly chopped fresh Italian parsley

sea salt and freshly cracked black pepper, plus Maldon sea salt for finishing

To make the vinaigrette, in a medium bowl whisk together the miso paste, almond butter, red curry paste, tamari or soy sauce, mirin or sweetened rice vinegar, unseasoned rice vinegar, chile pepper flakes, and garlic with the water until emulsified. Season with salt and pepper, if needed, and transfer to a glass jar. Store for up to 5 days in the refrigerator, and bring to room temperature before assembling the salad.

If using a large variety eggplant, you may need to "sweat" it to remove any bitterness. Place the quarters in a colander, and liberally salt each piece. Allow to sit for about 30 minutes, rinse well, and dry completely before roasting. Japanese eggplant, or a smaller variety, doesn't need this treatment.

To roast the zucchini and eggplant, preheat the oven to 425°F, and line two baking sheets with parchment paper.

Toss the zucchini with 1 tablespoon of the grapeseed oil, and season with salt and pepper. Bake for 15 minutes, flesh side down, until golden and beginning to soften.

Toss the eggplant with the remaining 2 tablespoons of grapeseed oil, and season with salt and pepper. Roast for 15 minutes, flesh side down, then turn each quarter over and roast for another 10 minutes, or until golden and soft in the center.

Allow the vegetables to cool slightly before slicing them on the bias into ½-inch pieces.

To assemble the salad, toss the eggplant, zucchini, and beans with the desired amount of vinaigrette in a large bowl. Serve on individual plates, garnish with fresh mint and parsley, and season with Maldon sea salt and pepper, if desired.

Cauliflower Salad
with Tuscan Kale Pesto

1–2 cloves garlic, roughly chopped

½ cup raw almonds

1 bunch Tuscan kale, ribs removed, and leaves roughly torn (about 3 cups)

½ cup nutritional yeast or ¼ cup Parmesan cheese, plus extra for garnish

1 teaspoon maple syrup, grade B

3 tablespoons fresh lemon juice, divided

¾ cup, plus 2 tablespoons extra virgin olive oil, divided

4 cups finely chopped white cauliflower florets (about 1 large head)

4 cups finely chopped purple cauliflower florets (about 1 large head)

4 large carrots, peeled and shaved with a vegetable peeler

3 cups finely torn red leaf lettuce

3 cups cooked chickpeas

1 cup thinly sliced celery

½ cup roughly chopped raw pistachios

¼ cup roughly chopped Italian parsley

sea salt and freshly cracked black pepper, plus Maldon sea salt to finish

This salad is beautiful without being overly fussy or contrived. It's also very low maintenance, and even gets better after sitting for 15 to 20 minutes, which allows the garlicky kale pesto to infuse every nook with flavor. My young son assisted in the creation of the pesto recipe. His little fingers neatly tore each kale leaf off the stalk—and he's very generous with garlic and salt. A sign that he's most definitely mine.

NOTE: *Nutritional yeast is inactive yeast, without leavening ability, derived from sugar cane and beet molasses. It imparts an umami, cheese-like flavor, along with copious amounts of B vitamins and other vital nutrients to the pesto. Parmesan cheese can easily stand in, if nutritional yeast is not your thing.*

Pulse the garlic and almonds in a food processor until roughly chopped. Add the kale, and pulse until well combined. Next, add the yeast or cheese, maple syrup, and 1 tablespoon of the lemon juice. With the motor running, stream in ½ cup plus 2 tablespoons of the olive oil, along with sea salt and black pepper, until combined but still somewhat chunky. Add more salt and pepper, if needed. Transfer the pesto to a glass jar, and refrigerate for up to 5 days.

To assemble the salad, place the two kinds of cauliflower and the carrots, lettuce, chickpeas, celery, pistachios, and parsley in a large serving bowl. Drizzle the remaining ¼ cup of olive oil and 2 tablespoons of lemon juice over the top. Add the desired amount of pesto, and season with Maldon sea salt and black pepper. Toss until well combined. Sprinkle extra nutritional yeast or cheese over the top just before serving.

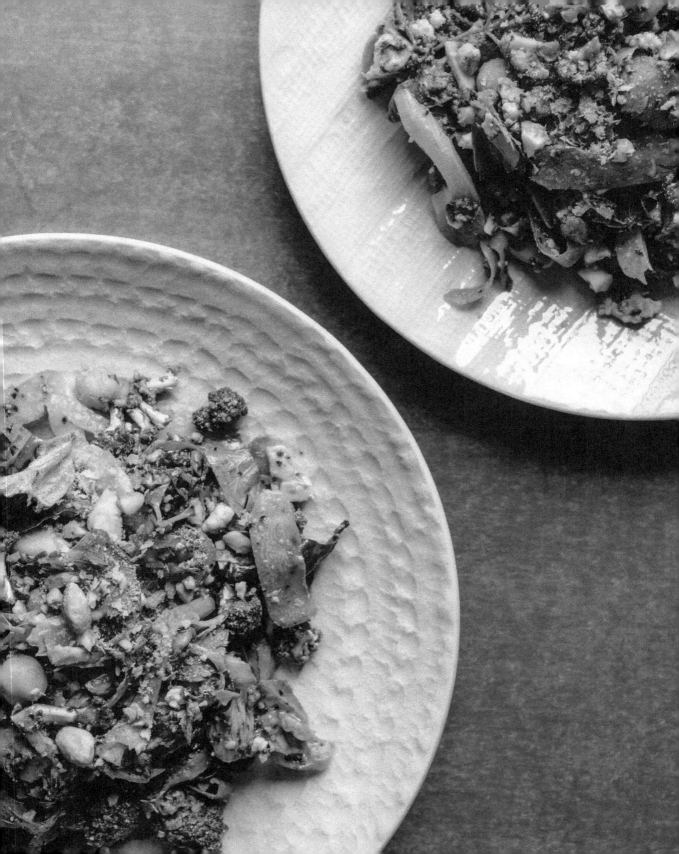

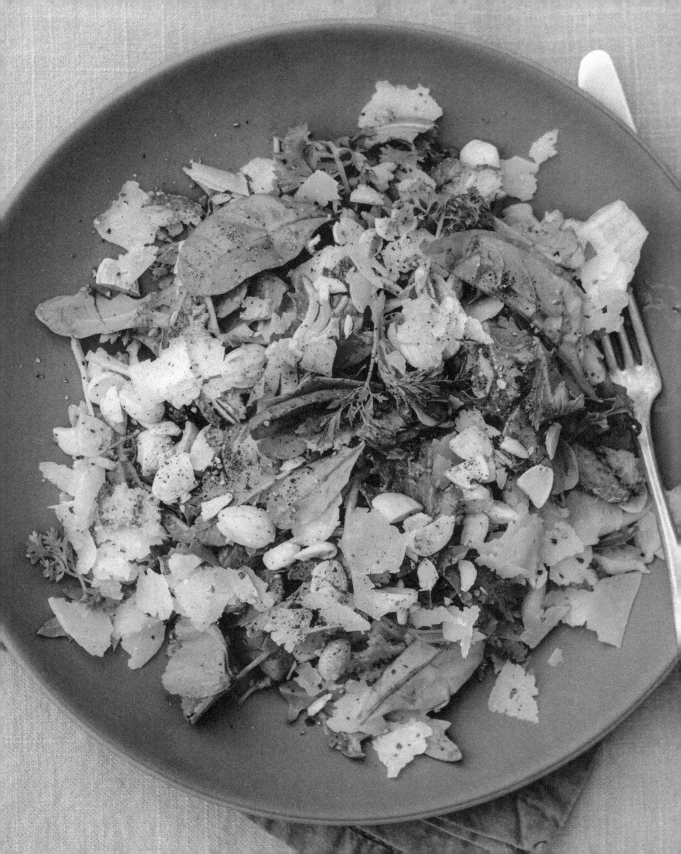

Spanish Bread Salad
with Smoky Quince–Black Pepper Vinaigrette

I've been fortunate to eat at some inspiring restaurants in my life. A meal at Arzak in San Sebastián, Spain, tops the list. The food that came out of that kitchen, and the endless creativity, were inspiring beyond words. Not one sense was left untouched. Even still, some of the simplest combinations of ingredients can be equally inspiring. Membrillo (quince paste) and manchego cheese is a classic Spanish pairing that does just that.

For the vinaigrette, place the membrillo or marmalade, mustard, vinegar, coriander, black peppercorns, garlic, and smoked paprika in a food processor, and pulse to combine. Slowly stream in ½ cup of the olive oil until well combined, and season with salt. Transfer to a glass jar and refrigerate for up to a week.

Place a grill pan over medium-high heat. Brush each piece of bread with the remaining 1 tablespoon of olive oil, and grill for about 1 minute per side, or until grill marks form and the bread begins to get crispy on the outside. Remove from the heat, and set aside to cool. Roughly tear into bite-size pieces once cool.

Drain the fennel on a towel, and pat to remove excess water. Arrange the bread, almonds, manchego, fennel, and greens on a large serving platter or on individual plates. Serve with the vinaigrette on the side. Sprinkle with Maldon sea salt and cracked pepper, if desired.

SERVES 4

2 tablespoons membrillo (quince paste) or orange marmalade

1 tablespoon, plus 1 teaspoon stone-ground mustard

¼ cup apple cider vinegar

2 teaspoons whole coriander, toasted and finely ground

2 teaspoons whole black peppercorns, finely ground

2 cloves garlic

½ teaspoon smoked paprika

½ cup, plus 1 tablespoon extra virgin olive oil

8 pieces of sourdough bread, thinly sliced

2 cups fresh fennel, thinly sliced (held in ice water until ready to use)

1 cup toasted and salted Marcona almonds, roughly chopped

¾ cup thinly shaved manchego cheese

4 cups arugula

4 cups mâche or other peppery green

sea salt and freshly cracked black pepper, plus Maldon sea salt for finishing

Warm Mushroom and Tofu Salad
with Chile-Lime Vinaigrette

SERVES 4

¾ cup tamari or soy sauce

1 tablespoon red chile flakes

1 clove garlic, finely diced

juice of 2 limes

2 tablespoons finely grated lemongrass

1 teaspoon maple syrup, grade B

¼ cup, plus 2 tablespoons grapeseed oil, divided

1 (10-ounce) block firm tofu, sliced into quarters lengthwise

5 cups cleaned, roughly sliced mushrooms

¾ cup finely diced shallot (about 1–2 medium shallots)

2 cups cooked barley

4 scallions, finely sliced on the bias

1 cup roughly torn mint, plus extra for garnish

1 cup roughly torn cilantro, plus extra for garnish

1½ tablespoons Sticky Rice Powder (page 83)

sea salt and freshly cracked black pepper

Mushrooms are abundant in Thailand. Northeastern Thai, or Isaan, cuisine formed the inspiration for this warm, rich salad. The traditional dish, het paa naam tok (forest mushroom salad), provides all the flavor notes that make food from this region so irrefutably delicious. For the mushrooms, choose at least two varieties, such as shiitake, oyster, king trumpet, or any other meaty mushroom.

Prepare the vinaigrette by adding the tamari or soy sauce, chile flakes, garlic, lime juice, lemongrass, maple syrup, and 3 tablespoons of the grapeseed oil to a medium bowl. Whisk until well combined. Season with salt and pepper, if necessary. Set aside until ready to use.

In a large cast-iron or other heavy skillet over medium heat, add 1 tablespoon of the grapeseed oil, and swirl to coat the pan. Cook the tofu squares for about 2 minutes per side, or until golden and crisp on the edges. Remove from the pan, and tent with foil to keep warm.

Wipe out the skillet, and add the remaining 2 tablespoons of grapeseed oil over medium-high heat. Swirl to coat the pan, and add the mushrooms. Sauté for 5 to 6 minutes, or until the mushrooms begin to soften and turn golden around the edges. Add the shallot and barley, and cook for another 1 to 2 minutes.

Turn off the heat, and add the vinaigrette, scallions, mint, cilantro, and sticky rice powder. Gently combine in the skillet, and season with salt and pepper, if desired. Serve on individual plates and garnish with additional fresh herbs, if desired.

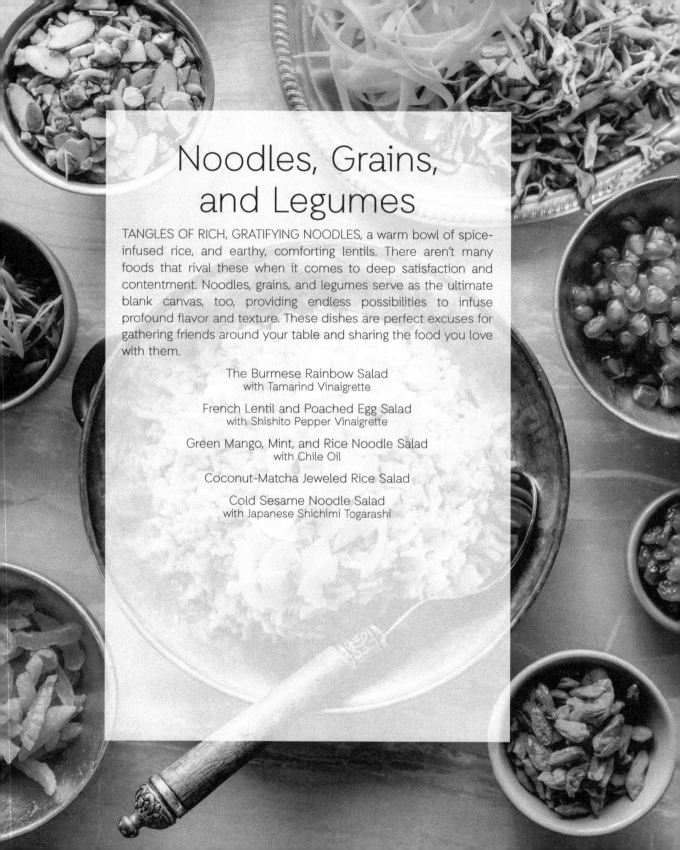

Noodles, Grains, and Legumes

TANGLES OF RICH, GRATIFYING NOODLES, a warm bowl of spice-infused rice, and earthy, comforting lentils. There aren't many foods that rival these when it comes to deep satisfaction and contentment. Noodles, grains, and legumes serve as the ultimate blank canvas, too, providing endless possibilities to infuse profound flavor and texture. These dishes are perfect excuses for gathering friends around your table and sharing the food you love with them.

The Burmese Rainbow Salad
with Tamarind Vinaigrette

French Lentil and Poached Egg Salad
with Shishito Pepper Vinaigrette

Green Mango, Mint, and Rice Noodle Salad
with Chile Oil

Coconut-Matcha Jeweled Rice Salad

Cold Sesame Noodle Salad
with Japanese Shichimi Togarashi

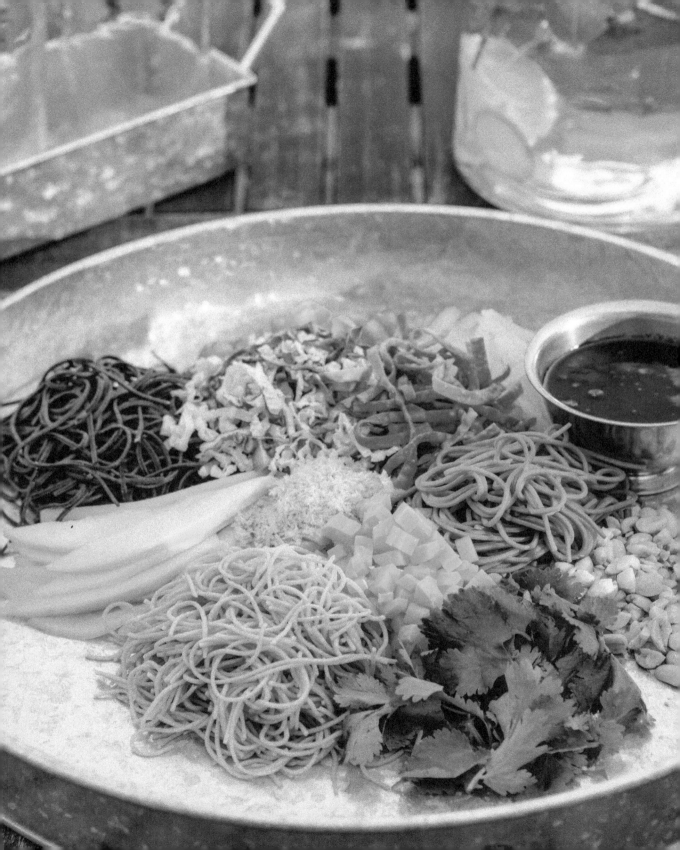

The Burmese Rainbow Salad
with Tamarind Vinaigrette

The tea leaf salad has earned icon status for very good reason. Texturally exciting, bold, and undeniably unique are attractive qualities. The rainbow salad, or let thohk sohn, is also a popular dish in the Burmese repertoire. Artfully composed, with a multitude of distinct and harmonious ingredients, it rivals the tea leaf salad, many people might say.

NOTE: *Indigenous to Africa, tamarind is a sour fruit that grows in large, clustered brown pods on the tamarind tree. Its most familiar use is in pad thai preparation. Although the flavor of tamarind is unique, 2 tablespoons of fresh lime juice may be substituted. For the noodles, I recommend using two to three different varieties such as brown rice noodles, black rice noodles, and green tea noodles.*

In a medium saucepan over medium-high heat, warm the grapeseed oil until just bubbling. Add the wonton strips, and fry until golden brown, about 2 to 3 minutes, stirring occasionally. Remove from the oil, season with salt, and allow to drain on paper towels.

To make the vinaigrette, whisk together the tamarind paste, chickpea flour, fish sauce, and maple syrup in a medium bowl. Slowly stream in the garlic oil until emulsified, and season with salt and pepper. Transfer to a glass jar, and refrigerate for up to a week.

Cook the noodles separately, drain, and rinse with cold water. Set aside until ready to assemble the salad.

Toss the crispy garlic, noodles, papaya, tomato, carrot, cabbages, bell pepper, cilantro, and peanuts, along with the dried shrimp and black garlic, if using, with the desired amount of vinaigrette in a large serving bowl. Season with salt and pepper, and garnish with extra cilantro before serving.

SERVES 4

2 cups grapeseed oil

8 wonton sheets, thinly cut into ⅛-inch strips

1 tablespoon tamarind paste

2 tablespoons Toasted Chickpea Flour (page 84)

3 tablespoons fish sauce

1 tablespoon maple syrup, grade B

¾ cup Garlic Oil (page 89)

4–5 cups various cooked noodles

¾ cup julienned green papaya

½ cup finely diced tomato

1 cup julienned carrot

1 cup finely shredded purple cabbage (about half of a small head)

1 cup finely shredded Napa cabbage (about half of a small head)

½ cup thinly sliced yellow bell pepper

¾ cup finely chopped cilantro, plus extra for garnish

½ cup roughly chopped Roasted Peanuts (page 84)

1 tablespoon ground dried shrimp (optional)

2 cloves black garlic, finely diced (optional, see page 91)

sea salt and freshly cracked black pepper

French Lentil and Poached Egg Salad
with Shishito Pepper Vinaigrette

SERVES 4

1½ cups French green lentils, rinsed and picked through for debris

1 bay leaf

½ cup, plus 1 tablespoon extra virgin olive oil, divided

¼ cup, plus 2 tablespoons grapeseed oil, divided

1 pint (about 1½ cups) shishito peppers, rinsed and stems removed

1 tablespoon tahini (sesame seed paste)

1 tablespoon unseasoned rice vinegar

zest and juice of 1 lemon

¼ teaspoon maple syrup, grade B

½ cup, plus 1 tablespoon filtered water

10–12 small sweet Italian peppers, stems and seeds removed, sliced into quarters

4–5 cloves garlic, thinly sliced lengthwise

4 large eggs

1 tablespoon apple cider vinegar

4 cups frisée (French curly endive) or other mild green lettuce, roughly chopped

6–8 slices of bacon, cooked and torn into small pieces (optional)

1 teaspoon ground Espelette pepper

sea salt and freshly cracked black pepper, plus Maldon sea salt for finishing

Thanks to their firmer texture, French green lentils, or lentilles du Puy, are the ideal base for hearty salads. They're often referred to as the caviar of lentils, due to the volcanic soil they're grown in producing an elegant, mineral-rich flavor. The traditional French salad, salade Lyonnaise, composed of bitter greens, crispy bacon and barely cooked eggs, was the inspiration for this recipe. This modern interpretation incorporates a tangy vinaigrette made with charred Japanese shishito peppers. Also, if you can find them, Jimmy Nardello sweet Italian peppers, originating in Southern Italy, work well in this recipe. The Slow Food organization has placed them in their international "Ark of Taste" directory, not only for their rich, unique flavor, but also because these peppers run the risk of becoming extinct.

NOTE: *Espelette pepper originates from the sun-drenched village of Espelette in Southern France. It's a prized and robust pepper that's slightly sweet and smoky. If you can't find the ground powder, substitute paprika or cayenne.*

In a large saucepan, add the lentils, and cover with filtered water (at least 4 to 5 inches above the lentils). Add the bay leaf, and bring to a boil over medium-high heat. Reduce the heat to a simmer, add a pinch of salt, and simmer for 20 to 25 minutes, or until the lentils are tender but still retain their shape. Drain, and set aside to cool. Once cool, gently toss with 1 tablespoon of the olive oil, and season with salt and pepper, if necessary. Set aside while you assemble the remaining ingredients.

For the vinaigrette, add 1 tablespoon of the grapeseed oil to a large cast-iron or other heavy skillet over medium-high heat. Once the oil is shimmering, add the shishito peppers. Cook undisturbed for 1 to 2 minutes, or until the peppers begin to char. Stir, and allow to cook for another 1 to 2 minutes, or until the peppers have blistered and begun to soften. Remove from the heat, and season with salt.

Once the peppers are cool, transfer them to a blender, and add the tahini, rice vinegar, lemon zest and juice, maple syrup, and filtered water. Pulse to combine. With the motor running, stream in the remaining ½ cup of olive oil. Season with salt and pepper, and transfer to a glass jar. Use immediately or refrigerate for up to a week.

Place the same pan used for the shishito peppers over medium-high heat and add 1 tablespoon of the grapeseed oil. Add the sweet Italian peppers and cook for 1 to 2 minutes, or until they begin to char. Shake the pan and allow the peppers to blister further, about another 1 or 2 minutes, until they begin to soften. Remove and slice into ⅛-inch strips.

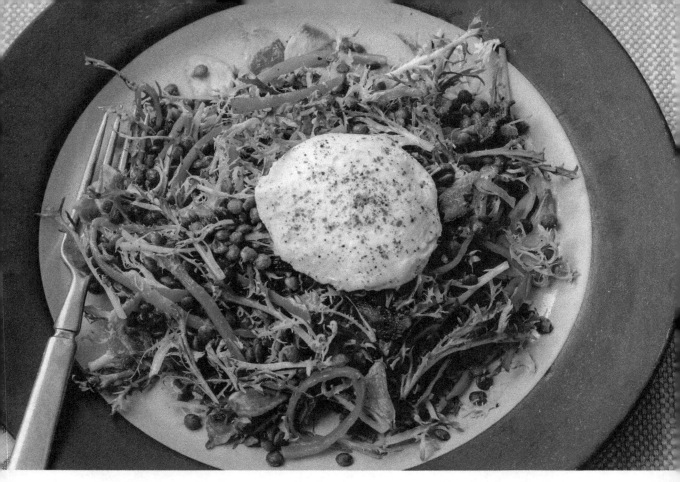

In a large saucepan over medium heat, bring the remaining ¼ cup of grapeseed oil to a low boil. Add the thinly sliced garlic and simmer, shaking occasionally, for about 4 to 5 minutes, or until the garlic turns golden brown. Remove with a slotted spoon, and drain on a paper towel. Transfer the garlic oil to a glass jar for another use.

To poach the eggs, use the freshest eggs you can find. Fill a medium saucepan halfway with water, and bring to a gentle boil. Add the apple cider vinegar to help the protein in the whites coagulate. Gently crack the eggs into the simmering water, allowing room between each egg. Cook for 4 to 6 minutes, depending on how runny you like your yolk. Remove from the water with a slotted spoon, and place on a towel to allow the excess water to drain.

This salad might be best assembled in individual portions, but you decide. Plate the lentils, peppers, fried garlic, frisée, poached egg, and bacon, if using. Sprinkle Espelette pepper on the egg, and Maldon sea salt and black pepper on the remainder of the salad. Serve with the vinaigrette on the side.

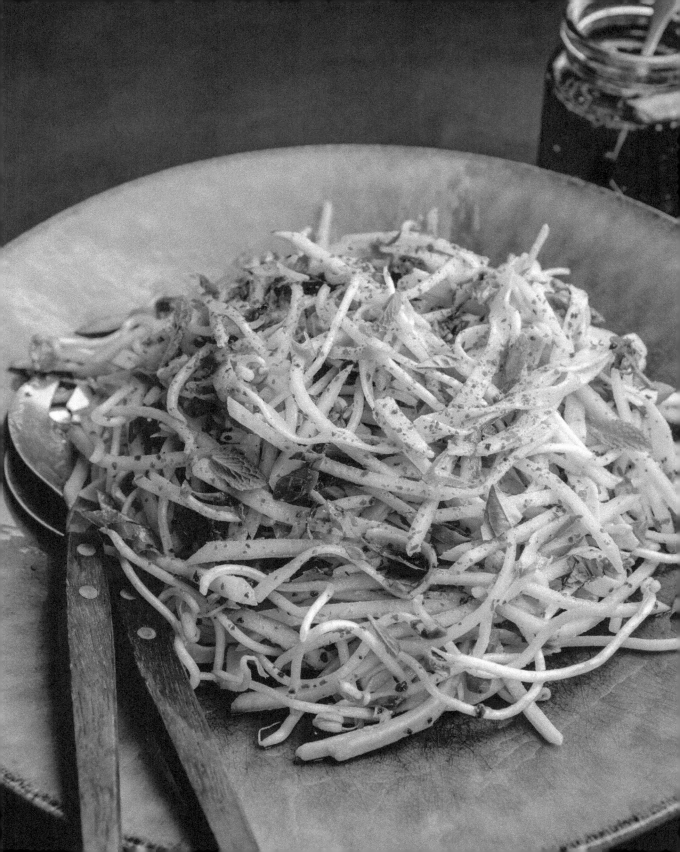

Green Mango, Mint, and Rice Noodle Salad
with Chile Oil

Green mango is a prized ingredient in Burmese cooking. Used more like a vegetable than an unripe fruit, it is hard and slightly sour when green. After a quick marinade in lime juice and salt, it takes on a new life and brings deep, bright flavor to the composed dish.

NOTE: *The mango has two seasons, spring/summer and fall/winter, allowing a year-round supply. When shopping for green mango, look for fruit that's firm and dense, and shows the least visible signs of ripening (pink, red, and orange hues).*

In a medium bowl, toss the sliced mango with the juice of 1 lime and a generous pinch of sea salt. Allow to sit for 10 minutes while you cook the noodles according to the package instructions. Drain, rinse the noodles with cold water to prevent sticking, and shake off the excess water before assembling the salad.

In a large serving bowl, add the noodles, green mango, mung bean sprouts, scallions, mint, basil, and 3 tablespoons of the chickpea flour. Drizzle the chile oil and fish sauce over the top, and toss to combine. Garnish with the chile flakes, the remaining 1 tablespoon of chickpea flour, and the remaining lime, quartered into wedges, and Maldon sea salt right before serving.

SERVES 4

1 green mango, peeled and sliced into very thin matchsticks

2 limes, divided

8 ounces brown rice pad thai noodles

1 (9-ounce) package mung bean sprouts

5–6 scallions, thinly sliced on the bias

½ cup roughly torn fresh mint

¼ cup roughly torn fresh basil

¼ cup Toasted Chickpea Flour (page 84), divided

¼ cup Chile Oil (page 88)

1 tablespoon fish sauce

1 tablespoon chile flakes

sea salt, plus Maldon sea salt for finishing

Coconut-Matcha Jeweled Rice Salad

SERVES 4-6

2 cups brown basmati rice, soaked in filtered water overnight

2 tablespoons grapeseed oil, divided

1 cup finely diced shallot (about 3 medium shallots)

1 clove garlic, finely diced

3 whole cloves

3-inch piece of Ceylon cinnamon stick

2 cups coconut milk

3 cups filtered water

1½ teaspoons matcha powder

1½ cups dried fruit (diced mango, apricots, cranberries, and goji berries are good choices)

1 cup golden raisins

½ teaspoon ground coriander

1 cup roughly chopped raw pistachios

½ cup raw slivered almonds

¼ cup raw seeds (pumpkin, sunflower, and hemp are good choices)

2 cups finely shredded purple cabbage (about 1 small head)

2 cups finely shredded carrots (about 3 large carrots)

1 cup pomegranate seeds

1 cup unsweetened coconut flakes

¼ cup finely chopped scallion

1 tablespoon orange zest (optional)

¼ cup good-quality extra virgin olive oil

sea salt and freshly cracked black pepper, plus Maldon sea salt for finishing

Iranian jeweled rice is traditionally created in Persian kitchens for weddings and other special occasions, fulfilling much the same role as tea leaf salad does in Myanmar. The original version is pigmented with saffron and is ultra-decadent, with copious amounts of butter and spices. Infused with coconut milk and antioxidant-rich matcha green tea, this lightened-up version requires some advanced preparation, but is a stunning addition to any celebration.

Drain and rinse the rice, shaking the strainer to remove any excess water. Add 1 tablespoon of the grapeseed oil to a large saucepan or Dutch oven over medium heat. Cook the shallot, garlic, cloves, and cinnamon stick for 1 to 2 minutes, stirring occasionally, until fragrant. Add the rice, and stir to combine. Add the coconut milk, filtered water, and matcha powder. Stir to combine, and bring to a boil. Once boiling, reduce the heat to low, and simmer, covered but slightly cracked open, for 40 to 45 minutes. If the rice is fully cooked but hasn't absorbed all the liquid, it's perfectly fine to drain. Remove the cloves and cinnamon stick, and allow to cool uncovered. Fluff the rice with a fork, and season with salt and pepper.

While the rice is cooking, in a medium skillet over medium heat, add the remaining 1 tablespoon of grapeseed oil. Add the dried fruit, raisins, and coriander. Stir occasionally until the fruit begins to soften, about 3 to 4 minutes. Season with salt and pepper, and transfer to a plate to cool. In the same skillet, toast the pistachios, almonds, and seeds over medium heat for about 2 to 4 minutes, and transfer to another plate to cool.

Arrange the rice, fruit mixture, nuts and seeds, cabbage, carrots, pomegranate seeds, coconut flakes, scallion, and orange zest, if using, on a large serving platter or on individual plates. Drizzle with the best-quality extra virgin olive oil you can find, and sprinkle with finishing salt and freshly cracked black pepper, if desired. Toss thoroughly at tableside to combine.

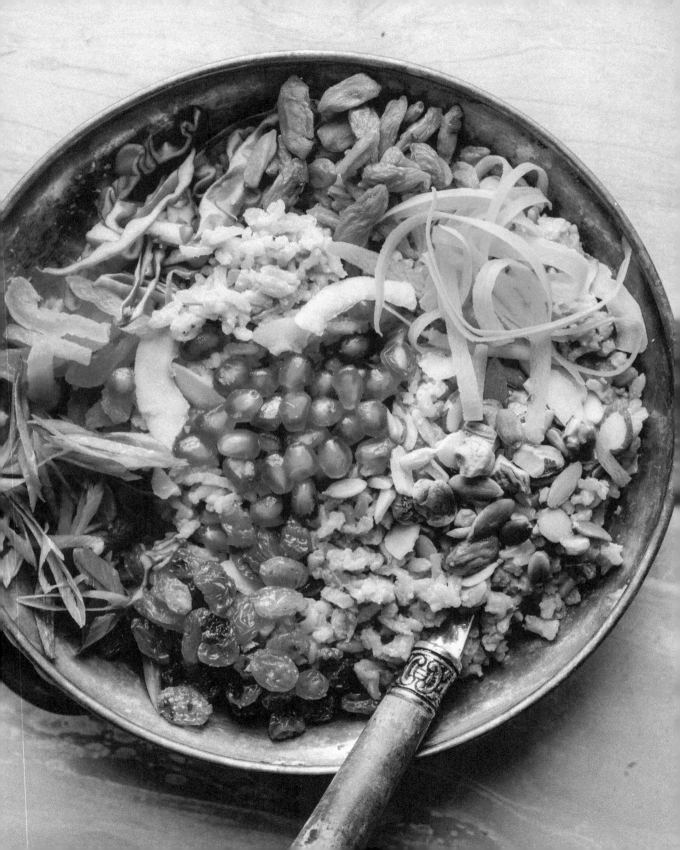

Cold Sesame Noodle Salad
with Japanese Shichimi Togarashi

SERVES 4

4 (3 x 2-inch) segments of orange peel, white pith removed

1 tablespoon red chile flakes

1 tablespoon ground Sichuan pepper

1 tablespoon raw white sesame seeds

½ tablespoon raw black sesame seeds

½ tablespoon raw chia seeds

3 tablespoons raw hemp seeds

½ sheet dried untoasted seaweed (nori), ground

2 teaspoons Earl Grey tea leaves, ground

4 cups roughly chopped broccolini (about 2 bunches)

2 tablespoons grapeseed oil

14 ounces brown rice fettuccini

6 cups packed spinach, roughly chopped

1 large yellow bell pepper, julienned

1 large orange bell pepper, julienned

¼ cup, plus 1 tablespoon toasted sesame oil

sea salt and freshly cracked black pepper, plus Maldon sea salt for finishing

On its own, this salad is clean and bright. What gives it immense depth of flavor is the Japanese shichimi togarashi, or seven spice. Coarsely ground chiles and other nutrient-dense seeds, spices, and citrus peels are to credit for the power of this condiment, traditionally found on the shelves of herbal medicine providers. My version of the spice blend incorporates a few non-traditional ingredients, like chia seeds and crushed Earl Grey tea leaves. Any leftover blend is excellent sprinkled on grilled meats and vegetables or a simple bowl of steamed rice. Consider adding grilled chicken or shrimp to the salad for a protein-dense version.

Dry the orange peels by leaving them on parchment paper at room temperature overnight or by placing them on a small baking sheet in a 200°F oven for 15 to 20 minutes, until fully dehydrated.

Grind the dried peels in a spice mill or with a mortar and pestle and place in a medium bowl. Add the chile flakes, Sichuan pepper, four types of seeds, seaweed, and tea, and stir to combine. Transfer to a glass jar and refrigerate for up to a month.

Next, preheat the oven to 425°F. Toss the broccolini with the grapeseed oil, salt, and pepper. Roast on a parchment-lined baking sheet for 15 to 20 minutes, or until the edges just begin to char. Remove from the oven, and allow to cool.

Cook the noodles according to the package instructions, adding the spinach during the last minute of cooking. Drain, rinse with cold water, and shake off the excess water before transferring to a large bowl. Add the broccolini, bell peppers, sesame oil, salt, and pepper (and additional protein, if using). With clean hands, gently toss until well combined. Serve in individual bowls, garnishing with the spice blend and Maldon sea salt before serving.

Fish and Shellfish

WHEN PREPARED WELL, seafood can be the ultimate in luxury. That said, finding an ultra-fresh resource matters. Since their inception in 2007, community-supported fishery (CSF) programs have grown in number—good news for those who don't live on or near the coast, or have a reputable fishmonger nearby. Much like the community-supported agriculture (CSA) model, CSFs foster a positive relationship between the consumer and commercial fishing by providing high-quality seafood while supporting marine ecosystems.

If I had to choose, I'd say this is my favorite section. Not only because I adore fresh seafood and the many health benefits it offers, including omega-3s and an extensive list of essential nutrients, but because these salads are so vibrant. And decadent. They make me feel happy to be alive. I'm pretty certain that's reason enough.

Sea Scallop, Pickled Ginger, and Avocado Salad
with Chamomile-Citrus Vinaigrette

Romaine on Romaine
with Garlic Shrimp and Saffron-Ginger Vinaigrette

Cider Smoked Salmon and Toasted Rye Salad
with Pickled Onion and Thyme Cream

Grilled Calamari Salad
with Spicy Kimchi Vinaigrette

Seared Tuna and Dragon Fruit Salad
with Basil Oil and Lemon Salt

Warm Black Cod and Shiitake Mushroom Salad
with Whipped Avocado

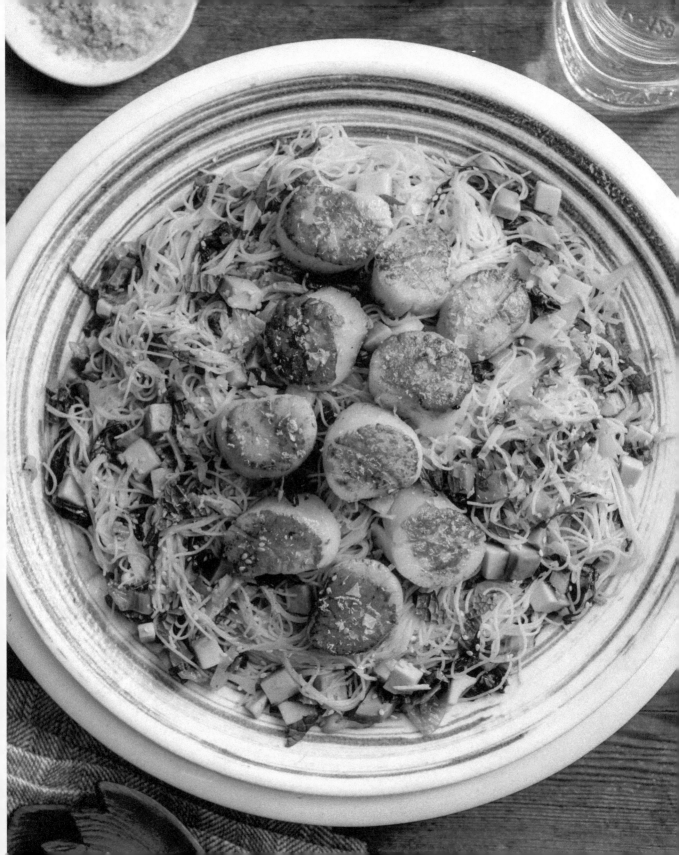

Sea Scallop, Pickled Ginger, and Avocado Salad
with Chamomile-Citrus Vinaigrette

Living within a mile of the New England coast as a child had its perks. Ultra-fresh seafood was commonplace at family gatherings, and briny sea scallops quickly rose to the top of my list of favorites. This salad is inspired by those memories in tandem with the sushi I've grown to love as an adult on the West Coast.

SERVES 4

½ cup brewed chamomile tea, plus 1 teaspoon whole chamomile flowers, finely ground

2 tablespoons Greek yogurt

1 tablespoon, plus 1 teaspoon grapefruit zest, divided

¼ teaspoon ground turmeric

1 tablespoon lemon zest

1 tablespoon lemon juice

¾ cup, plus 1 tablespoon grapeseed oil

6 ounces maifun (angel hair) brown rice noodles

1 tablespoon extra virgin olive oil

1 large romaine heart, quartered

12 large sea scallops, cleaned and dried, side muscle removed

2 medium avocados, finely diced

2½ tablespoons finely diced Pickled Ginger (page 87)

¼ cup roughly torn fresh mint, plus extra small leaves for garnish

¼ cup toasted sesame seeds

sea salt and freshly cracked black pepper, plus 1 tablespoon Maldon sea salt

For the vinaigrette, in a medium bowl, combine the brewed tea, the yogurt, 1 tablespoon of the grapefruit zest, and the turmeric, lemon zest, and lemon juice. Slowly whisk in ¾ cup of the grapeseed oil until emulsified, and season with salt. Refrigerate for up to 5 days. Shake well before using.

To make the finishing salt, combine the ground tea with the remaining 1 teaspoon of grapefruit zest and 1 tablespoon of Maldon sea salt, and set aside.

Cook the noodles according to the package instructions, rinse with cold water, and drain. Set aside until ready to assemble the salad.

Drizzle the olive oil over the romaine hearts, and season with salt and pepper. Preheat the grill, or cast-iron skillet, to medium-high heat, and cook the romaine for about 4 to 6 minutes, until the edges begin to char and the romaine softens, turning once. Remove from the heat, and allow to cool before chopping finely.

To get the best sear, blot any excess water from the scallops with paper towels. Season with salt and pepper. In a large, heavy skillet over high heat, add the remaining 1 tablespoon of grapeseed oil until shimmering. When the pan is very hot, add the scallops, being careful not to overcrowd. Cook for about 2 minutes per side, or until golden and bouncy to the touch. Remove from the heat, and set aside to cool.

Plate the noodles, romaine, avocado, ginger, mint, and sesame seeds, and drizzle on the desired amount of vinaigrette. Toss to combine. Add the scallops, and sprinkle the finishing salt over the top. Serve with extra vinaigrette, if desired.

Romaine on Romaine
with Garlic Shrimp and Saffron-Ginger Vinaigrette

SERVES 4

2 pounds wild shrimp or prawns, peeled and deveined, tails left intact or removed

1 tablespoon grapeseed oil

3 cloves garlic, finely diced

2 large romaine hearts, finely chopped, with 4 whole outer green leaves set aside

1-inch piece of ginger, peeled and roughly chopped

1 medium shallot, roughly chopped

2 tablespoons coconut vinegar

½ teaspoon saffron threads

2 tablespoons crème fraîche or Greek yogurt

½ teaspoon maple syrup, grade B

¼ cup, plus 1 tablespoon extra virgin olive oil, divided

2 Granny Smith apples, sliced into ¼-inch matchsticks (reserved in cold water with a squeeze of lemon to prevent oxidation)

2 large avocados, diced (with a squeeze of lemon to prevent oxidation)

¼ cup sesame seeds, toasted

sea salt and freshly cracked black pepper, plus Maldon sea salt for finishing

Often placed in the same lonely category as iceberg lettuce, romaine contains an impressive amount of vitamins and minerals. One in particular, the trace mineral manganese, is found in abundance, offering significant antioxidant protection, increased collagen production, and improved skin integrity.

NOTE: *Coconut vinegar, the by-product of coconut blossom extraction is loaded with amino acids, prebiotics, and vitamins. Champagne vinegar can be substituted for the coconut vinegar, although it does not provide the same nutrient boost.*

In a medium bowl, toss the shrimp with the grapeseed oil, garlic, sea salt, and pepper. Refrigerate for at least an hour, or overnight.

To make the vinaigrette, place the four reserved romaine leaves, ginger, shallot, vinegar, saffron, crème fraîche or yogurt, maple syrup, and ¼ cup of the olive oil in a blender. Season with salt and pepper, and blend until smooth. Transfer to a glass jar, and refrigerate for up to 5 days. The color will be most vibrant if the vinaigrette is used immediately, however.

Next, preheat your grill, grill pan, or heavy skillet over medium-high heat, and cook the shrimp for approximately 2 minutes per side, or until pink and opaque. Remove from the heat, and toss with the remaining 1 tablespoon of olive oil. Add salt and pepper, if necessary. Once cool, leave whole or slice into bite-size pieces.

Toss the chopped romaine, apple, avocado, shrimp, and sesame seeds with the desired amount of vinaigrette in a large bowl. Serve on individual plates and garnish with Maldon sea salt and freshly cracked black pepper, if desired.

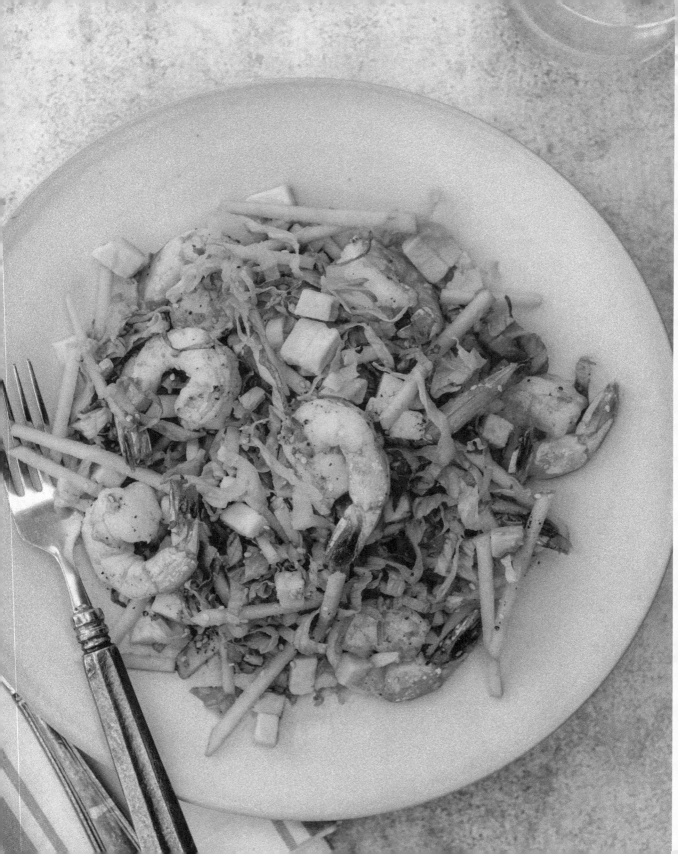

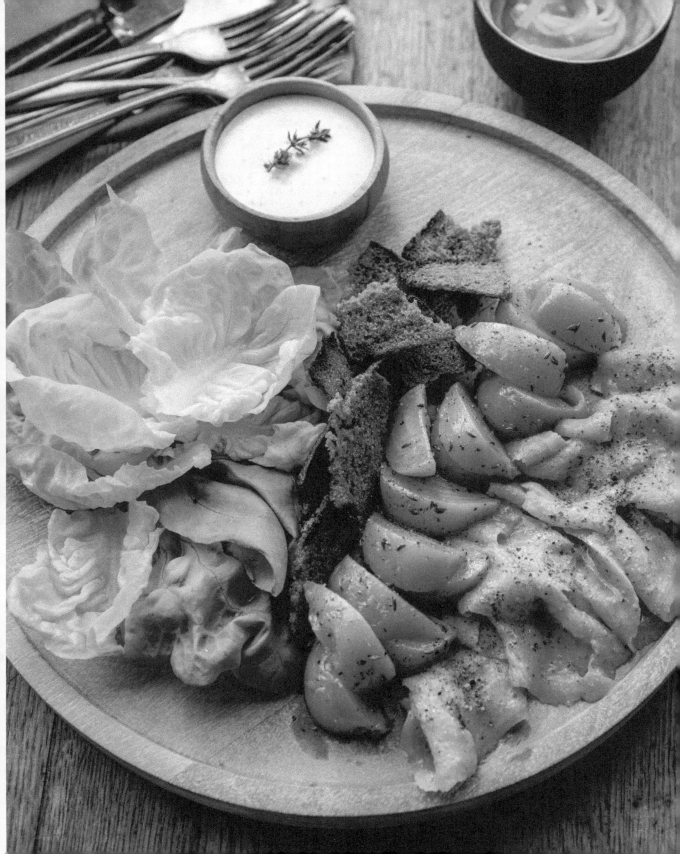

Cider Smoked Salmon and Toasted Rye Salad
with Pickled Onion and Thyme Cream

Years ago, I spent several weeks in London with my hilarious friend Chris as a tour guide. Adventuring through the narrow, picturesque streets, you never know quite what you'll find. There's soul and a sense of life pulsing through every quaint corner of this city. My favorite part of each day was when we'd tuck into a neighborhood pub for a cider. Those days seemed to unfold effortlessly. The cider, stone-ground mustard, and truffle oil marinade for the salmon is as effortless and thrilling as that unforgettable trip.

SERVES 4

1 cup apple cider

¼ cup stone-ground mustard

1 teaspoon white truffle oil (optional)

16 ounces wild smoked salmon

6 medium golden beets, cleaned, both ends trimmed

1 tablespoon grapeseed oil

1 cup crème fraîche or Greek yogurt

1 teaspoon finely chopped fresh thyme leaves

8 slices dense rye bread, each about ¼ inch thick

¼ cup, plus 1 tablespoon Caraway Oil (page 88), divided

½ cup Pickled Red Onion (page 86)

2 heads butter lettuce, torn into bite-size pieces

sea salt and freshly cracked black pepper

In a medium bowl, whisk together the cider, mustard, sea salt, pepper, and truffle oil, if using. Slice the salmon into about 2 x 3-inch pieces. Gently toss to combine in the marinade, cover tightly, and refrigerate for 1 hour.

Preheat the oven to 400°F. Place the beets on a large piece of parchment paper, and drizzle with the grapeseed oil. Wrap the paper around the beets, folding the edges to secure them, and place on a baking sheet. Bake on the middle rack of the oven for 35 to 45 minutes, or until a fork inserted into the middle easily pierces the beets. Remove from the oven, and allow to cool before peeling and slicing into quarters.

In a medium bowl, combine the crème fraîche or yogurt with the thyme, and season with salt and pepper. Cover and refrigerate the thyme cream for up to 5 days.

To make the toasted rye, brush the bread on both sides with 1 tablespoon of the caraway oil, and place on a grill pan or other heavy skillet, over medium-high heat. Cook for 2 to 3 minutes per side, or until grill marks form and the bread is crispy. Once cool, tear into bite-size pieces.

On a large platter or on individual plates, arrange the marinated salmon, beets, rye bread, pickled red onion, and lettuce. Drizzle the lettuce and beets with the remaining ¼ cup of caraway oil. Season with salt and pepper, if desired. Serve the thyme cream on the side.

Grilled Calamari Salad
with Spicy Kimchi Vinaigrette

SERVES 4

¼ cup unseasoned rice vinegar

2 tablespoons toasted sesame oil

1¼ cups roughly chopped Spicy Kimchi (page 90), divided

1 tablespoon filtered water

½ cup, plus 2 tablespoons grapeseed oil, divided

3 pounds calamari, tubes and tentacles, cleaned and dried thoroughly with paper towels

4 cups finely shredded purple cabbage (about 1 medium head)

4 cups unpeeled, finely diced English cucumber (about 1 large)

4–6 cups watercress

1½ tablespoons lemon zest

½ cup roughly chopped fresh chives

¼ cup roughly torn, packed fresh basil

1 tablespoon red chile flakes

sea salt and freshly cracked black pepper, plus Maldon sea salt for finishing

Referred to as calamari in the Mediterranean, squid is a popular food in many regions of the world because it is inexpensive and versatile. For some, especially those who aren't familiar with it, calamari can seem unapproachable. Still, I urge you to give it a chance. When prepared well, calamari is an extraordinary ingredient. Just make sure to buy ultra-fresh calamari and ask your fishmonger to clean it for you to save time. For the best sear, thoroughly dry the calamari before lighting your grill. If you still can't get behind the idea, shrimp can stand in, too.

NOTE: *If you're not up for the task of making kimchi from scratch, you'll find many excellent varieties sold today.*

For the vinaigrette, add the rice vinegar, sesame oil, 1 cup of the kimchi, filtered water, salt, and pepper to a blender, and pulse until well combined. With the motor running, slowly stream in ½ cup of the grapeseed oil until emulsified. Transfer to a glass jar, and refrigerate for up to a week.

Preheat the grill, grill pan, or heavy skillet over high heat. Toss the calamari with salt, pepper, and the remaining 2 tablespoons of grapeseed oil. If the squid pieces are on the smaller side, you may want to place them in a fish basket or utilize one of the indoor cooking methods so they don't fall through the grates. Place the calamari tubes on the hot grill, and weigh them down with a heavy skillet. Allow to cook, undisturbed, for 1 or 2 minutes, or until grill marks form. Turn over for another 1 or 2 minutes. Remove from the heat, and slice into thin strips.

To cook the tentacles, place them directly on the grates, and cook for 1 to 2 minutes per side, or until the ends become slightly charred, then turn over and cook for another 1 or 2 minutes. Roughly chop or leave whole.

Toss the calamari, cabbage, cucumber, watercress, lemon zest, and chives with the desired amount of vinaigrette in a large serving bowl. Garnish with fresh basil, the remaining ¼ cup of kimchi, chile flakes, Maldon salt, and pepper.

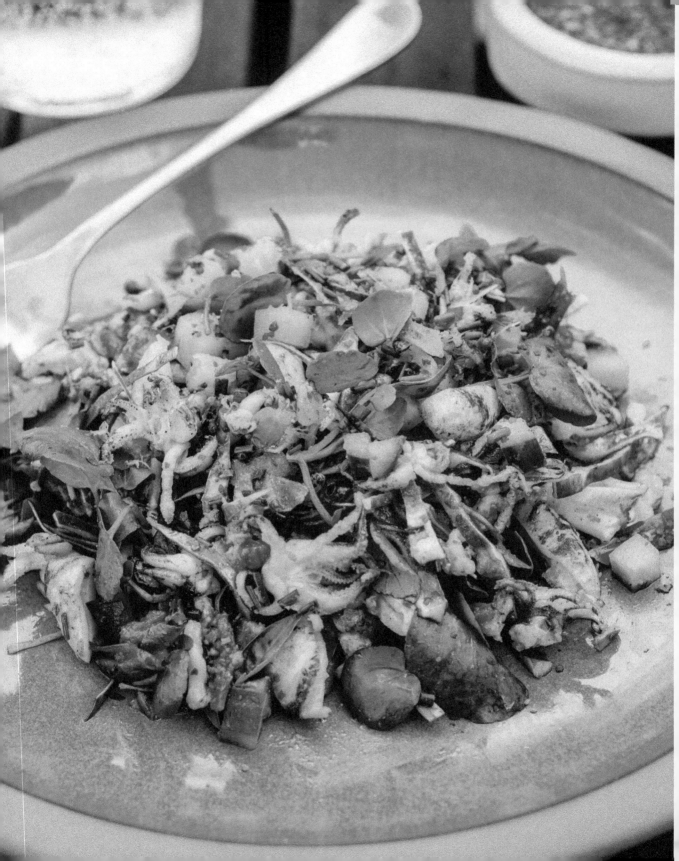

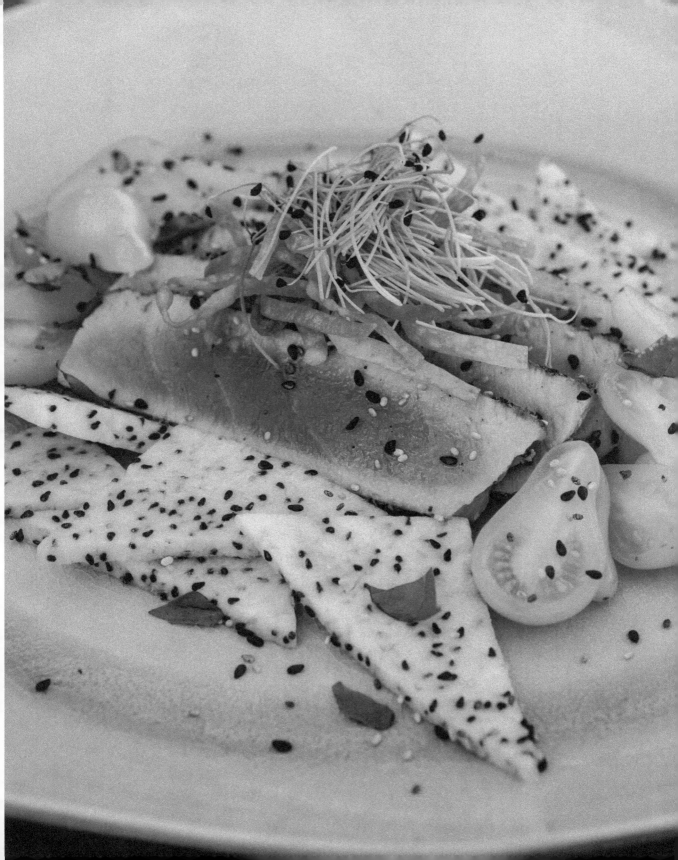

Seared Tuna and Dragon Fruit Salad
with Basil Oil and Lemon Salt

Grown throughout Southeast Asia, the spiky tropical dragon fruit, or pitaya, is a playful match for the fennel and black pepper–crusted tuna in this salad. The fruit's interior is either white or ruby and is dotted with edible black seeds. Dragon fruit, found year-round, tastes like a cross between pear, kiwi, and watermelon.

For the basil oil, prepare a medium bowl of ice water. Bring a pot of water to a boil, and blanch the basil leaves for 10 to 15 seconds. Remove and quickly submerge them in the ice water for 1 to 2 minutes. Drain and place on a towel to dry, gently squeezing to remove excess water. Place in a blender with the garlic clove, olive oil, and a pinch of sea salt, and puree until well combined. Pour through a fine-mesh strainer, gently pushing on the solids with the back of a spoon to extract the oil. Place in a glass jar. Use immediately, or refrigerate for up to 5 days. Bring to room temperature before using because the oil may solidify.

To make the salt, combine the lemon zest and Maldon salt in a small ramekin, and set aside until ready to use.

Next, in a medium saucepan over medium-high heat, heat 1 cup of the grapeseed oil until it is shimmering. Carefully drop one wonton strip into the oil to test the temperature. If tiny bubbles surround it, the rest are ready to go in. Use a slotted spoon to slowly turn and move the wonton strips around in the oil occasionally. They're done when light golden brown. Remove and place on a towel-lined plate to drain. Sprinkle with sea salt, and set aside until ready to assemble.

For the tuna, drizzle ½ tablespoon of the grapeseed oil over the steaks, and sprinkle with the ground fennel. Season with sea salt and a generous amount of cracked black pepper.

Place a cast-iron pan or heavy skillet over high heat, and add the remaining 1 tablespoon of grapeseed oil, swirling to coat the pan. Once the pan is very hot, add the tuna and cook for about 2 minutes per side, depending on the thickness. This cooking time is recommended for a tuna steak approximately 2 inches thick. The goal is to get a golden sear on each side while retaining a pink interior. Remove from the heat, and allow to cool for a few minutes before thinly slicing against the grain.

On a large platter or on individual plates, arrange the tuna, tomatoes, dragon fruit, and sesame and chia seeds. Scatter torn fresh basil and microgreens, if using, over the top. Serve the basil oil and lemon salt on the side. Allow any leftover lemon salt to sit out overnight for the zest to dry, then transfer it to an airtight container for up to two weeks.

SERVES 4

- 2 cups tightly packed fresh basil leaves, plus extra for garnish
- 1 clove garlic
- 1 cup extra virgin olive oil
- 1 tablespoon lemon zest
- 1 tablespoon Maldon sea salt, plus extra for finishing
- 1 cup, plus 1½ tablespoons grapeseed oil, divided
- 10 wonton wrappers, thinly sliced into 1/8-inch strips
- 2 pounds sushi-grade tuna steaks
- 1 tablespoon roughly ground fennel seeds
- 3 cups halved golden cherry tomatoes
- 2 medium dragon fruits, sliced in half, peeled, and sliced into bite-size pieces (watermelon or kiwi are good substitutes)
- 2 tablespoons raw white sesame seeds
- 2 tablespoons raw black chia seeds or black sesame seeds
- microgreens, for garnish (optional)
- sea salt and freshly cracked black pepper

Warm Black Cod and Shiitake Mushroom Salad
with Whipped Avocado

SERVES 4

2 pounds black cod fillets

2½ tablespoons, plus 1 teaspoon white miso paste, divided

¼ cup grapeseed oil, divided

½ cup filtered water

1 large yellow onion, quartered and thinly sliced

4 cups thinly sliced shiitake mushrooms (roughly 1½–2 pounds)

2 cups diced avocado (about 2 large avocados)

¼ cup unseasoned rice vinegar

1 teaspoon maple syrup, grade B

¼ cup, plus 2 tablespoons extra virgin olive oil, divided

4 cups watercress or other peppery green

sea salt and freshly cracked black pepper

Black cod is easy to love. Full of beneficial omega-3 fats, sustainably harvested, and oh so buttery when cooked well, it has a lot going for it. When marinated in miso paste, whether overnight or only for an hour, it morphs into a classic Japanese-inspired meal, fit for a weeknight or to impress a table full of your favorite guests.

Remove any pin bones from the fillets, and slice the fish into equal portions, about 4 to 5 inches long, and place them in a sealable container. In a medium bowl, combine 2½ tablespoons of the miso paste with 1 tablespoon of the grapeseed oil and the filtered water. Pour over the fish, and cover tightly. Marinate in the refrigerator overnight, or at least for a couple of hours.

Next, caramelize the onion. In a medium sauté pan over medium-high heat, add 1 tablespoon of the grapeseed oil. When the oil begins to shimmer, add the onion. Once the onion begins to turn a golden color, reduce the heat to low. Cook for 30 to 40 minutes, stirring frequently, until the onion becomes soft and a deep caramel color develops. Remove from the heat, and season with salt and pepper. Keep warm until ready to use.

Remove the fish from the refrigerator 20 to 30 minutes prior to cooking.

In a large, heavy skillet over medium-high heat, add the remaining 2 tablespoons of grapeseed oil. Once the oil begins to shimmer, add the mushrooms and allow them to sit, undisturbed, for a minute or two. Stir occasionally, and cook until soft and golden around the edges, about 5 or 6 minutes. Season with salt and pepper, and keep warm while you compose the rest of the dish.

To make the whipped avocado, place the avocado, remaining 1 teaspoon of miso paste, rice vinegar, maple syrup, sea salt, and pepper in a food processor, and pulse to combine. Slowly stream in ¼ cup plus 1 tablespoon of the olive oil, and set aside, covered, until ready to use.

To prepare the fish, preheat the broiler and line a baking sheet with aluminum foil. Shake off any excess miso marinade from the fish, and place on the sheet. Bake on the upper rack of the oven for 8 to 10 minutes, or until the edges begin to caramelize and crisp and the fish is somewhat firm to the touch.

To assemble the salad, toss the watercress with the remaining 1 tablespoon of olive oil, and lightly season with salt and pepper. Arrange the onion, mushrooms, watercress, and cod on a large serving platter or on individual plates. Because the miso can be salty, you probably won't need any finishing salt for this dish. Serve the whipped avocado on the side.

Chicken, Turkey, and Duck

A DEPENDABLE SOURCE OF HIGH-QUALITY PROTEIN, these salads are unique in their own ways. In this section, we'll make a trek from Myanmar to Mexico, Laos to Italy, and back around to Asia with a tea-crusted duck salad brought to life by copious amounts of finely ground smoky lapsang souchong tea. Plenty of golden turmeric, aromatic star anise, red curry paste, and fiery chiles are also incorporated, making these salads complex and intense, in all the right ways.

Lemongrass Chicken Salad
with Golden Vinaigrette

Chicken, Black Bean, and Charred Poblano Salad
with Pumpkin–Red Curry Vinaigrette

Garam Masala Turkey Salad
with Tamarind-Cranberry Agrodolce

Grilled Tamari-Ginger Chicken Salad
with Creamy Chive Vinaigrette

Tea-Crusted Duck and Mandarin Salad
with Star Anise–Black Pepper Vinaigrette and Tea Salt

Turkey Larb Salad

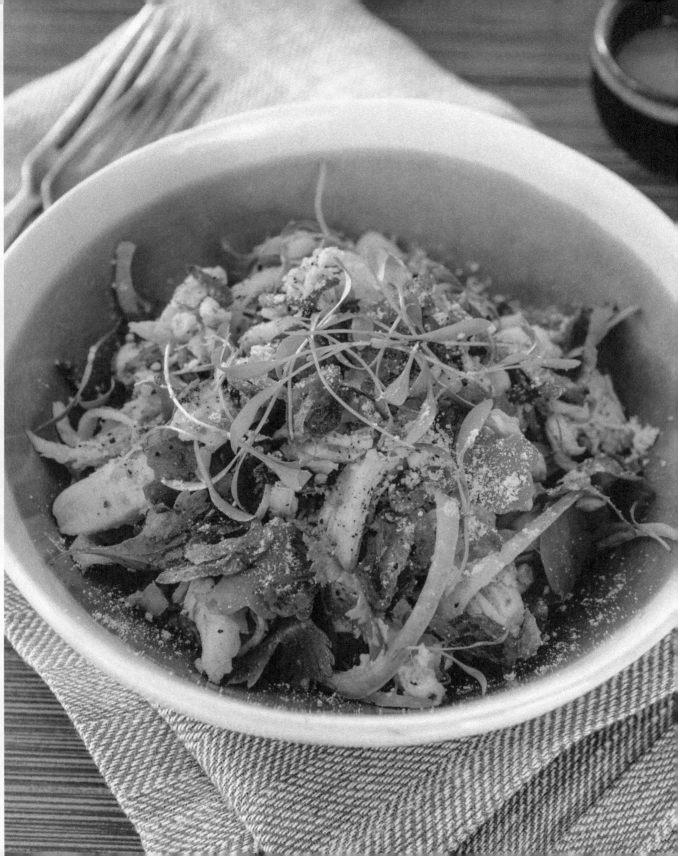

Lemongrass Chicken Salad
with Golden Vinaigrette

The golden temples of Myanmar inspired the use of turmeric as one of the key ingredients in this salad which displays a similar vibrant color. The first time I worked with turmeric, I walked around with yellow hands for days. This is why it's a highly coveted medicinal spice in many cuisines: potency.

NOTE: *If you can find micro–cilantro, use it, as it lends a subtler flavor and beautiful presentation to the finished dish.*

SERVES 4

2 tablespoons extra virgin olive oil

3 lemongrass stalks, tough outer layers removed, finely grated with a microplane (about 2 tablespoons)

1 teaspoon dried red chile flakes (Aleppo works well)

2 pounds bone-in, skinless chicken breast, poached and shredded into bite-size pieces

1 teaspoon ground turmeric

2 tablespoons fresh carrot juice

¼ teaspoon finely grated fresh ginger

3 tablespoons champagne vinegar or white wine vinegar

1 teaspoon maple syrup, grade B

½ cup Shallot Oil (page 89)

4 small shallots, finely diced and soaked in cold water for 20 to 30 minutes

¾ cup Crispy Shallots (page 89)

¾ cup fresh cilantro, finely chopped, plus extra for garnish

½ cup fresh mint, finely torn into pieces

¼ cup Toasted Chickpea Flour (page 84), divided

1 cup mâche or other peppery green

1 lemon, quartered

sea salt and freshly cracked black pepper, plus Maldon sea salt for finishing

To a medium skillet over medium heat, add the olive oil. Once it is shimmering, add the lemongrass and chile, and sauté for 1 to 2 minutes, or until soft and aromatic. Then add the shredded chicken, and season with salt and pepper. Toss to combine, remove from the heat, and allow to cool. The chicken mixture may be used immediately or refrigerated overnight.

For the vinaigrette, whisk together the turmeric, carrot juice, ginger, vinegar, and maple syrup. Slowly whisk in the shallot oil until well combined. Season with salt and pepper, and transfer to a glass jar. This vinaigrette is best used within a couple of days.

Toss the chicken, fresh and crispy shallots, cilantro, mint, 3 tablespoons of the chickpea flour, salt, and pepper with the desired amount of vinaigrette in a large bowl. Serve in individual bowls or on separate plates. To garnish, toss the mâche with 1 teaspoon of vinaigrette, and arrange over the top. Garnish with the remaining 1 tablespoon of the chickpea flour, Maldon salt, extra cilantro, and lemon wedges.

Chicken, Black Bean, and Charred Poblano Salad
with Pumpkin–Red Curry Vinaigrette

SERVES 4

2 teaspoons whole coriander, toasted

2 tablespoons, plus 1 teaspoon whole cumin seed, toasted, divided

1-inch piece of Ceylon cinnamon stick

¼ teaspoon smoked paprika

½ cup, plus 2 tablespoons pumpkin puree

2 cloves garlic, roughly chopped

1 tablespoon Thai red curry paste

¼ cup unseasoned rice vinegar

2 tablespoons mirin, or 2 tablespoons rice vinegar with 1 teaspoon maple syrup added

1 teaspoon maple syrup, grade B

¼ cup, plus 2 tablespoons extra virgin olive oil

2–3 pounds bone-in, skin-on chicken breasts

1 tablespoon grapeseed oil

2 large poblano peppers

2 cups cooked black beans

2 cups finely shredded purple cabbage (about 1 small head)

2 cups grated smoked mozzarella cheese (about 8 ounces)

¼ cup finely chopped chives

¼ cup finely chopped cilantro

¼ cup raw hemp seeds

sea salt and freshly cracked black pepper, plus Maldon sea salt for finishing

The poblano is a versatile, mild pepper originating from Puebla, Mexico. It is the star of the popular stuffed chile dish called chile rellenos. This salad is a healthier, deconstructed version loaded with protein-dense chicken and black beans, and featuring pumpkin–red curry vinaigrette for just the right amount of mellow heat.

NOTE: *Hemp seeds are a concentrated source of protein, omega fatty acids, minerals, and antioxidants. They are soft, with a mild nutty flavor. Toasted pine nuts are a good substitute if you don't have hemp seeds.*

To make the vinaigrette, grind the coriander, 1 tablespoon plus 1 teaspoon of the cumin, and the cinnamon stick in a spice grinder until fine. In a blender or food processor, combine the spices with the paprika, pumpkin, garlic, red curry paste, unseasoned rice vinegar, mirin or sweetened rice vinegar, and maple syrup. With the motor running, slowly stream in the olive oil until emulsified, and season with salt and pepper. Transfer to a glass jar, and refrigerate for up to 5 days.

For the chicken, preheat the oven to 400°F, and line a baking sheet with parchment paper. Drizzle the grapeseed oil over each breast. Grind the remaining 1 tablespoon of cumin, and season with cumin, salt, and pepper. Bake for about 30 minutes, bone side down, or until the internal temperature registers at least 165°F. Remove from the oven, allow to cool, and shred the chicken. Set aside until ready to assemble the salad.

Place the poblano peppers over a direct flame (your hottest gas burner or grill). Carefully rotate with tongs until the peppers are completely blackened. Remove from the heat, and place in a paper bag or wrap in parchment paper for 10 to 15 minutes. The steam makes it easier to peel the skins. Once the peppers are cool, remove the skin. Don't worry if you can't remove all the charred bits. Leaving some intact lends a smoky flavor to the dish. Remove the stem and seeds, and slice into 1/8-inch strips. Season with salt and pepper.

To assemble, arrange the shredded chicken, peppers, beans, cabbage, cheese, herbs, and hemp seeds on a large platter or on individual plates. Season with Maldon sea salt and pepper, and serve the vinaigrette on the side.

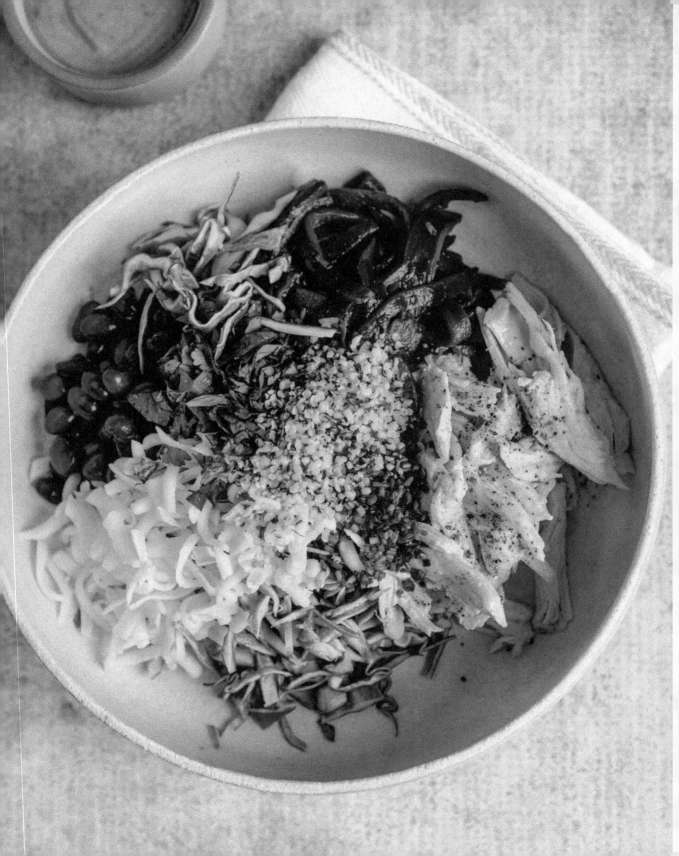

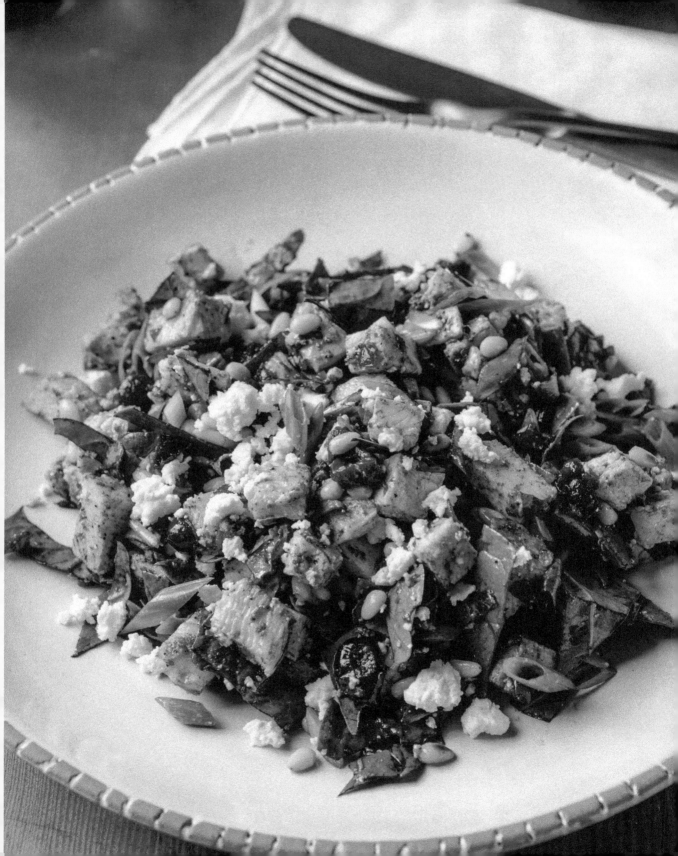

Garam Masala Turkey Salad
with Tamarind-Cranberry Agrodolce

This complex salad incorporates flavors from India and Italy and is a great use of leftover Thanksgiving turkey. Garam masala is a deeply flavorful spice mix containing cinnamon, nutmeg, cloves, cardamom, mace, coriander, cumin, and peppercorns. Typically used as a finishing spice in northern Indian and South Asian cuisines, the blend raises the internal temperature of the body and boosts metabolism.

NOTE: *Similar to a French gastrique, agrodolce is a jammy, sweet and sour condiment popular in Italian cuisine.*

Preheat the oven to 425°F. Rub 1½ tablespoons of the garam masala along with sea salt and pepper onto the turkey breast, distributing evenly. In a large cast-iron or other heavy skillet over medium-high heat, add the grapeseed oil. Once the oil is shimmering, place the turkey breast, skin side down, in the pan. Cook for about 4 minutes, or until golden. Turn the breast over, and transfer to the oven for another 20 to 25 minutes, or until the internal temperature reaches at least 165°F. Allow to cool before slicing into bite-size pieces.

For the agrodolce, whisk together the cranberries, shallot, rice vinegar, tamarind paste, garlic, chile pepper flakes, and maple syrup in a medium saucepan over high heat. Once boiling, season with salt and pepper, and lower to medium. Simmer for 10 to 12 minutes, or until reduced by about half, with a slightly syrupy consistency. Add the remaining ½ teaspoon of garam masala, and stir to combine. Remove from the heat, and transfer to a glass jar. The agrodolce may be refrigerated for up to a week.

Toss the turkey, pine nuts, feta, scallion, spinach, olive oil, and black pepper with the desired amount of agrodolce in a large bowl. Serve on individual plates and garnish with extra scallions.

SERVES 4

4 pounds bone-in, skin-on turkey breast

1½ tablespoons, plus ½ teaspoon garam masala, divided

1 tablespoon grapeseed oil

½ cup roughly chopped dried cranberries

2 tablespoons finely diced shallot

3 cups unseasoned rice vinegar

2 tablespoons tamarind paste (¼ cup lime juice may be substituted)

2 finely diced cloves garlic

1 pinch dried chile pepper flakes

¼ cup maple syrup, grade B

1 cup pine nuts, lightly toasted

¾ pound feta cheese

½ cup finely diced scallion, plus extra for garnish

4 cups roughly chopped spinach

¼ cup extra virgin olive oil

sea salt and freshly cracked black pepper

Grilled Tamari-Ginger Chicken Salad
with Creamy Chive Vinaigrette

SERVES 4

1 cup tamari

½ cup dry white wine

1 tablespoon grated ginger

1 tablespoon grated garlic

2 teaspoons fines herbes, divided

2 tablespoons grapeseed oil

3–4 boneless, skinless chicken breasts (about 2½ pounds), trimmed of excess fat, and sliced in half horizontally

1 large egg

1 medium shallot, roughly chopped

1 clove garlic

1 tablespoon Dijon mustard

2 tablespoons fresh lemon juice

½ teaspoon maple syrup, grade B

2 tablespoons champagne vinegar or white wine vinegar

¼ cup roughly chopped chives

1½ tablespoons toasted sesame oil

½ cup extra virgin olive oil

2½ cups thinly sliced sugar snap peas

2½ cups finely shredded Napa cabbage (about 1 medium head)

2 cups halved cherry tomatoes

1½ cups thinly shaved watermelon radish or other radish

¼ cup sesame seeds, toasted

1 lemon, cut into quarters

sea salt and freshly cracked black pepper, plus Maldon sea salt for finishing

For summer parties and lazy days by the pool, my mother would make endless batches of this chicken. Just about everyone asked for the recipe. Paired with a creamy vinaigrette that uses a protein-dense soft-boiled egg in lieu of mayonnaise, this salad is substantial and bright with a nod to Asian and French cuisine.

NOTE: *Tamari and soy sauce are both the result of fermented soybeans. Made with little to no wheat, tamari is a more deeply flavored, gluten-free alternative to soy sauce. Feel free to use soy sauce if you don't have tamari.*

In a medium bowl, whisk together the tamari, white wine, ginger, grated garlic, 1 teaspoon of the fines herbes, grapeseed oil, and black pepper. Add the chicken, turning several times to evenly coat it. Cover, and marinate in the refrigerator for 4 to 6 hours.

For the vinaigrette, cook the egg in boiling water for 7 minutes. Remove immediately, and rinse under cold water to stop the cooking. You should have a firm white and barely set yolk. Peel and place in a blender along with the shallot, garlic, mustard, lemon juice, maple syrup, and vinegar. Pulse to combine, scraping down the sides as you go. Add the chives, the remaining 1 teaspoon of fines herbes, salt, and pepper. With the motor running, stream in the toasted sesame oil and olive oil until emulsified. Transfer to a glass jar, and store in the refrigerator for up to 5 days.

Remove the chicken from the refrigerator and allow to sit at room temperature for 30 minutes. Next, preheat the grill to medium-high, or place an indoor grill pan or heavy-cast iron skillet over medium-high heat. Cook the chicken for about 2 to 3 minutes per side, until grill marks form and the internal temperature registers at least 165°F. If using a charcoal grill, create a two-zone fire, with all the coals on one side. Cook the chicken for about 2 minutes per side, then move it to the cool side of the grill, covered, to finish cooking through, if necessary.

Remove the chicken from the grill, and allow it to rest before slicing on the bias into bite-size pieces. The chicken can be made a day ahead and refrigerated overnight, if desired.

In a large serving bowl, toss the chicken, peas, cabbage, tomatoes, and radish with the desired amount of vinaigrette. Sprinkle with sesame seeds, Maldon sea salt, and black pepper. Serve with lemon wedges on the side.

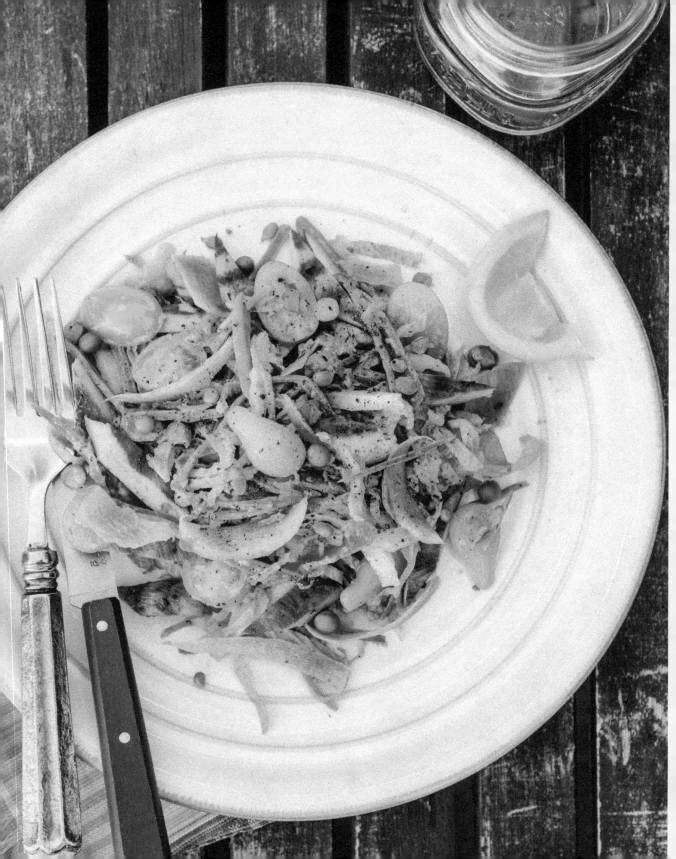

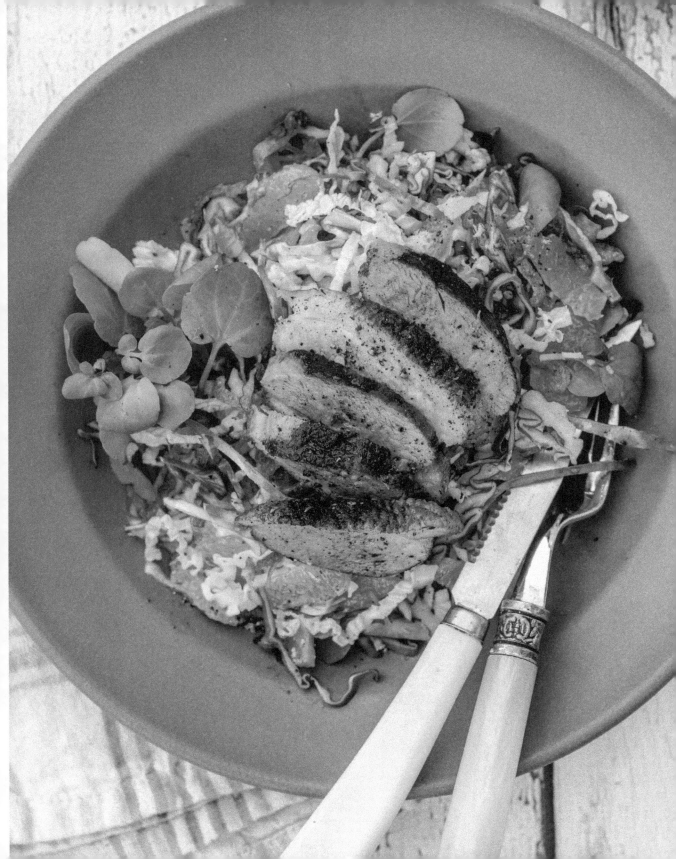

Tea-Crusted Duck and Mandarin Salad
with Star Anise–Black Pepper Vinaigrette and Tea Salt

Tea-smoked duck, or zhangcha duck, is an iconic and elaborate dish in southwestern China often reserved for celebrations. The traditional preparation includes a three-step process of hot smoking over black tea leaves and twigs of camphor, steaming, and then deep frying for an ultra-crisp result. This salad is dramatically simplified and lightened up, although the goal of bringing out deep, intense flavors remains.

SERVES 4

7 star anise pods

2 whole cloves

1½ teaspoons black peppercorns, divided

1 tablespoon whole coriander, toasted, divided

1 teaspoon fennel seed, toasted

zest and juice of 1 medium orange

1 tablespoon stone-ground mustard

1 clove garlic

1 teaspoon ground turmeric

1 teaspoon apple cider vinegar

1 teaspoon maple syrup, grade B

1 cup extra virgin olive oil

1 tablespoon, plus 2 teaspoons lapsang souchong black tea

1 tablespoon Maldon sea salt

2½ tablespoons grapeseed oil, divided

About 5–6 medium shallots, thinly sliced

2 duck breasts (about 1½–2 pounds)

2 cups mandarin orange segments

4 cups finely shredded Napa cabbage (about 1 large head)

4 cups finely shredded purple cabbage (about 1 large head)

2 cups watercress or other peppery green

2 tablespoons Pickled Ginger (page 87) (optional)

edible flowers, for garnish (optional)

sea salt and freshly cracked black pepper

For the vinaigrette, grind the star anise, cloves, ½ teaspoon of the black peppercorns, 1 teaspoon of the coriander, and fennel in a spice grinder until fine. Transfer to a blender, along with the orange zest, orange juice, mustard, garlic, turmeric, vinegar, and maple syrup. Pulse until well combined. With the motor running, stream in the olive oil until emulsified, and season with salt and additional black pepper, if desired. Transfer to a glass jar, and store in the refrigerator for up to 5 days.

Finely grind the tea and the remaining 2 teaspoons of coriander. Transfer 2½ teaspoons of the mixture to a small bowl, and combine with the Maldon sea salt. This is your finishing salt. Add the remaining 1 teaspoon of black peppercorns to the rest of the tea mixture, and grind until well combined. Set this aside for the rub.

Add 1½ tablespoons of the grapeseed oil to a medium skillet over medium heat. Add the shallot, and cook for 3 to 4 minutes, or until lightly caramelized and beginning to crisp. Season with salt and pepper, and transfer to a paper towel–lined plate to cool.

To prepare the duck, pat each breast with paper towels until very dry. This will create the best sear. Score the skin of each breast to prevent it from curling. Generously coat each breast with the tea rub, and season with salt and pepper. Preheat the oven to 400°F.

In a large cast-iron or other heavy ovenproof skillet over medium heat, add the remaining 1 tablespoon of grapeseed oil. Once the oil is shimmering, place each breast in the pan, skin side down. Allow to cook, undisturbed, for 4 to 5 minutes, or until a golden crust forms. Turn each breast over, and place the skillet in the preheated oven for another 8 to 10 minutes, or until the internal temperature of the breast registers 160° to 170°F (medium rare). Remove from the heat, and allow to cool for 5 to 10 minutes before slicing on the bias.

Toss the shallot, mandarin orange, cabbages, watercress, and pickled ginger with the desired amount of vinaigrette. Place on a large serving platter or on individual plates. Arrange the duck over the top, and drizzle additional vinaigrette. Garnish with tea salt and edible flowers, if using.

Turkey Larb Salad

SERVES 4

2 whole cloves

8 star anise pods

8 green cardamom pods, seeds removed and set aside for toasting

2 tablespoons cumin seeds

½ cup grapeseed oil

1 cup thinly sliced shallot (about 2–3 medium shallots)

1 cup red onion, quartered and thinly sliced

1 tablespoon whole Thai bird chiles

2 pounds ground turkey

¼ cup, plus 2 tablespoons fish sauce

½ cup lime juice (about 5–6 limes)

1 teaspoon maple syrup, grade B

2 cups roughly chopped mung bean sprouts

4 scallions, finely diced on the bias

2 cups finely shredded Napa or savoy cabbage (about 1 medium head)

¾ cup Sticky Rice Powder (page 83)

¼ cup roughly torn fresh mint, plus extra for garnish

¼ cup roughly chopped fresh cilantro, plus extra for garnish

¼ cup roughly torn fresh basil, plus extra for garnish

While some Laotians designate larb as the country's national dish, many argue that it is best described as a method, largely centered around finely chopped cooked or raw meat and an abundance of citrus, chiles, fresh herbs, and sticky rice powder. This version is best enjoyed warm or at room temperature. Also, instead of the salad being served in traditional lettuce cups, shredded cabbage is tossed in at the end to impart the signature texture and crunch.

NOTE: *Thai bird chiles can be found at specialty markets.*

In a medium skillet over medium heat, toast the cloves, star anise, cardamom seeds, and cumin seeds until fragrant, about 1 to 2 minutes. Once cool, grind into a fine powder, with a spice grinder or in a mortar and pestle, and set aside.

In a large skillet, warm the grapeseed oil over medium-high heat. Once the oil is shimmering, add the shallot, red onion, and chiles, stirring occasionally, until the ingredients begin to turn golden on the edges, about 5 minutes. Transfer to a towel-lined plate, and season with salt. If you don't want the finished dish extra spicy, consider removing the chiles at this point.

Add the turkey and ground spices to the same skillet, and cook until the turkey is no longer pink, about 4 to 5 minutes, mincing with a wooden spoon. Add the fish sauce, lime juice, and maple syrup, and stir to combine. Turn off the heat.

To the turkey mixture in the skillet, add the shallot mixture, mung beans, scallions, cabbage, sticky rice powder, and fresh herbs. Toss to combine, serve in individual bowls, and garnish with additional herbs.

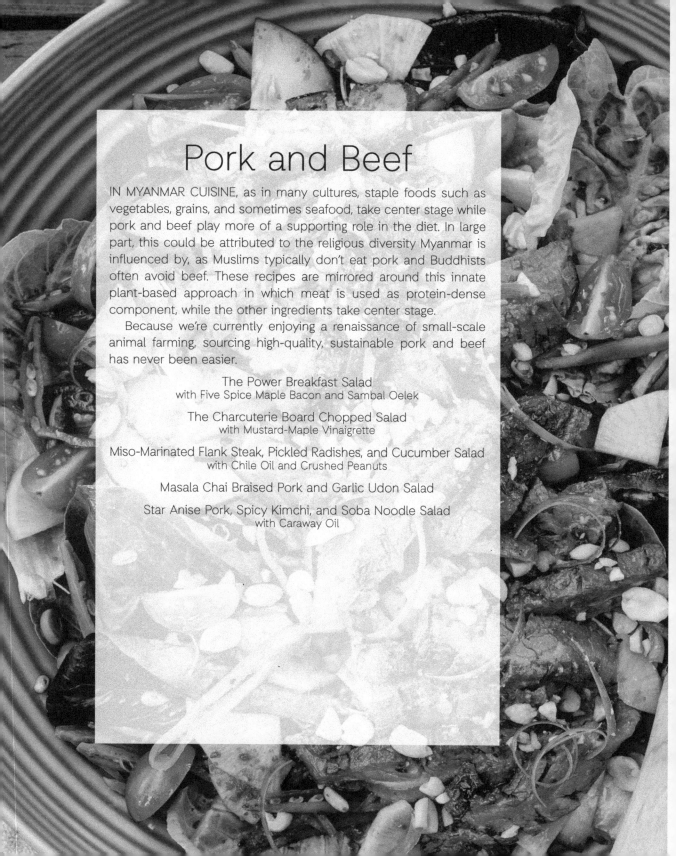

Pork and Beef

IN MYANMAR CUISINE, as in many cultures, staple foods such as vegetables, grains, and sometimes seafood, take center stage while pork and beef play more of a supporting role in the diet. In large part, this could be attributed to the religious diversity Myanmar is influenced by, as Muslims typically don't eat pork and Buddhists often avoid beef. These recipes are mirrored around this innate plant-based approach in which meat is used as protein-dense component, while the other ingredients take center stage.

Because we're currently enjoying a renaissance of small-scale animal farming, sourcing high-quality, sustainable pork and beef has never been easier.

The Power Breakfast Salad
with Five Spice Maple Bacon and Sambal Oelek

The Charcuterie Board Chopped Salad
with Mustard-Maple Vinaigrette

Miso-Marinated Flank Steak, Pickled Radishes, and Cucumber Salad
with Chile Oil and Crushed Peanuts

Masala Chai Braised Pork and Garlic Udon Salad

Star Anise Pork, Spicy Kimchi, and Soba Noodle Salad
with Caraway Oil

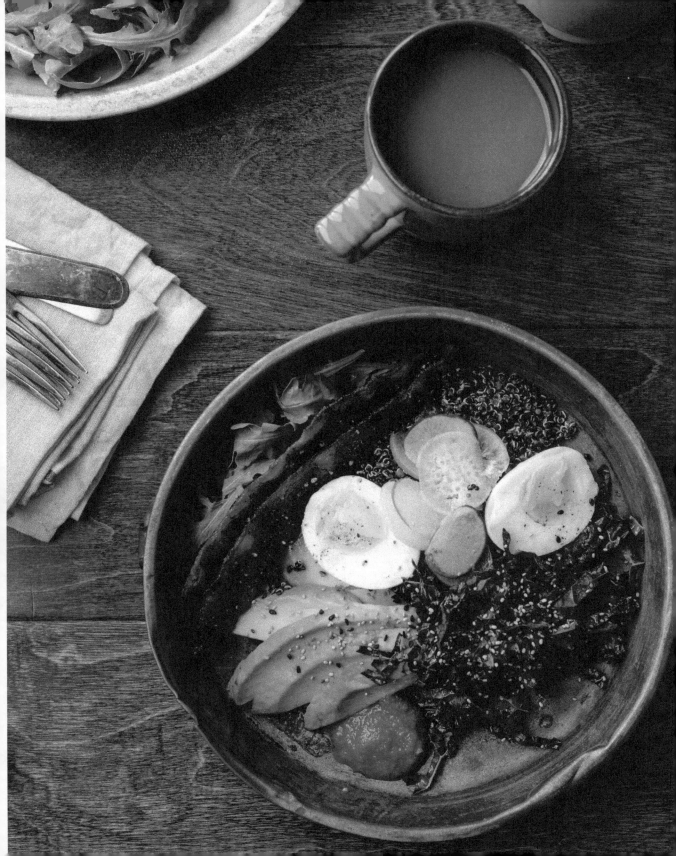

The Power Breakfast Salad
with Five Spice Maple Bacon and Sambal Oelek

Eating salad for breakfast may seem unconventional. However, the temptation to venture beyond the norm is irresistible in a world where Chinese five spice and maple bacon can come together with quinoa, greens, soft-boiled eggs, and fiery sambal oelek.

NOTE: *Sambal oelek is a Southeast Asian chile sauce. This version offers unadulterated heat with three simple ingredients: hot red chile peppers, rice vinegar, and salt. The active compound in the peppers, capsaicin, provides anti-inflammatory and antioxidant support while the vinegar is alkalizing. I recommend red Fresno, red serrano, or red jalapeño for the sambal oelek, and a variety of greens, such as kale and arugula, to provide a much-needed boost first thing in the morning.*

SERVES 4

- 12 red chile peppers
- 2 tablespoons unseasoned rice vinegar
- 8 ounces uncured bacon
- 2 teaspoons Chinese five spice
- 1 tablespoon maple syrup, grade B
- 4 large eggs
- 2 cups cooked quinoa, seasoned with salt and pepper
- 6 radishes, thinly shaved with a vegetable peeler or mandoline
- 4 cups greens
- 2 avocados, thinly sliced
- 1 tablespoon raw black sesame seeds
- 1 tablespoon raw white chia seeds
- sea salt and freshly cracked black pepper, plus Maldon sea salt for finishing

For the sambal oelek, slice the chiles in half, removing some seeds if you'd like your sauce less spicy. Roughly chop the chiles, and place in a food processor. Add the vinegar and sea salt, and pulse until a rough paste forms, scraping down the sides as you go. Transfer to a glass jar, and refrigerate for up to 2 weeks.

Preheat the oven to 400°F. Arrange the bacon slices on a parchment-lined baking sheet, and sprinkle with five spice and a generous amount of black pepper. Rub the spice mixture into each strip, and bake for 15 to 20 minutes, or until crisp. Place on a paper towel–lined plate, and drizzle with maple syrup. Keep warm until ready to assemble the salad.

Bring a medium pot of water to a rapid boil, and add the eggs. Allow to cook for 7 to 8 minutes, drain, and place under cold water to stop the cooking process. Peel the eggs, and slice them in half or quarters.

Toss the greens with extra virgin olive oil, and salt and pepper right before serving.

To assemble, place the quinoa, bacon, eggs, radish, greens, and avocado in individual bowls. Sprinkle the sesame seeds and chia seeds over the top, and season with Maldon sea salt and pepper, if desired. Serve the sambal oelek on the side.

The Charcuterie Board Chopped Salad
with Mustard-Maple Vinaigrette

SERVES 4

2 tablespoons finely diced shallot

2 tablespoons stone-ground mustard

2 tablespoons maple syrup, grade B

2 tablespoons apple cider vinegar

¼ cup, plus 3 tablespoons extra virgin olive oil, divided

1 bunch fresh sage, stems removed

¼ cup grapeseed oil

8–10 pieces of sourdough bread, thinly sliced

5–6 ounces mild salami, very thinly sliced

¼ cup roughly chopped olives

3 cups red leaf lettuce, roughly chopped

¼ cup raw or lightly toasted walnuts, roughly chopped

1–2 Anjou pears, thinly sliced (about 1½ cups)

¼ cup finely shaved pecorino cheese

sea salt and freshly cracked black pepper, plus Maldon sea salt for finishing

At the end of a long week, assembling a board brimming with cheese, meat, olives, and crusty bread is one of my favorite things to do for those I love. Of course, a great bottle of wine and plenty of cozy candlelight is in the mix, too. This casual, convivial approach to a meal provides time to linger, be present, and truly catch up. Inspired by those moments, this salad offers new flavor pairings to be discovered with each bite. The mustard-maple vinaigrette is the luscious constant that ties it all together. Any combination of olives will do, but I recommend Castelvetrano olives from Italy and Kalamata olives from Greece for this recipe.

For the vinaigrette, combine the shallot, mustard, maple syrup, and vinegar in a medium bowl. Slowly whisk in ¼ cup plus 2 tablespoons of the olive oil, and season with salt and pepper. Transfer to a glass jar, and refrigerate for up to a week.

To make crispy sage leaves, heat the grapeseed oil in a small skillet over medium-high heat. When the oil is shimmering, add 8 to 10 leaves at a time, and cook for about 3 to 5 seconds, or until crisp. Remove immediately with a slotted spoon, place on a paper towel–lined plate, and season with salt. Continue the same process with the remainder of the leaves.

Preheat the broiler, and place the sourdough slices on a parchment-lined baking sheet. Brush both sides with the remaining 1 tablespoon of olive oil, and broil for 1 to 2 minutes per side, or until golden and crisp. Allow to cool before tearing into bite-size pieces.

Arrange the salami, olives, lettuce, walnuts, and pears, along with the bread and sage on a large platter or on individual plates, and season with salt and pepper, if desired. This salad can be served deconstructed with the vinaigrette on the side, or tossed with the vinaigrette right before serving.

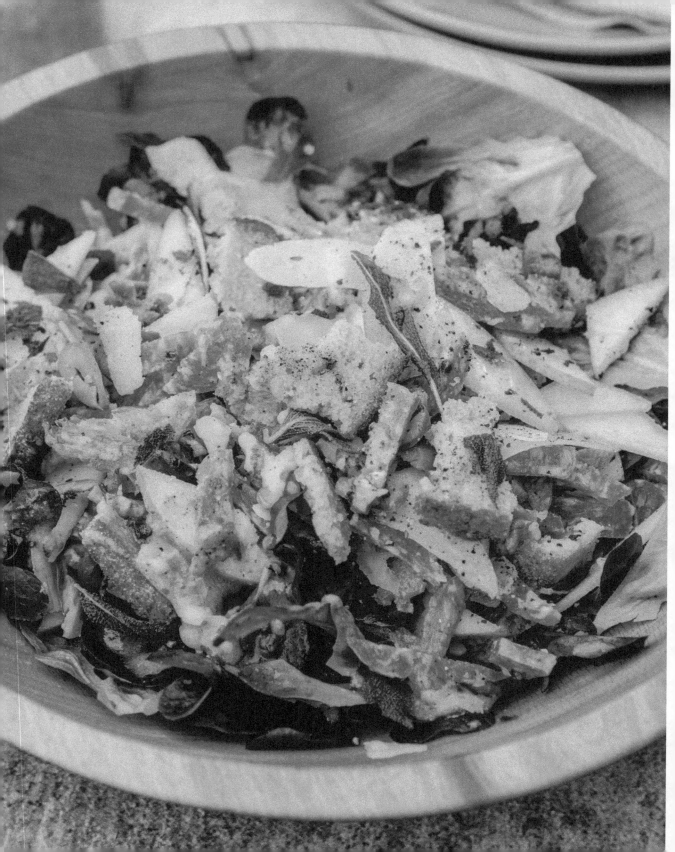

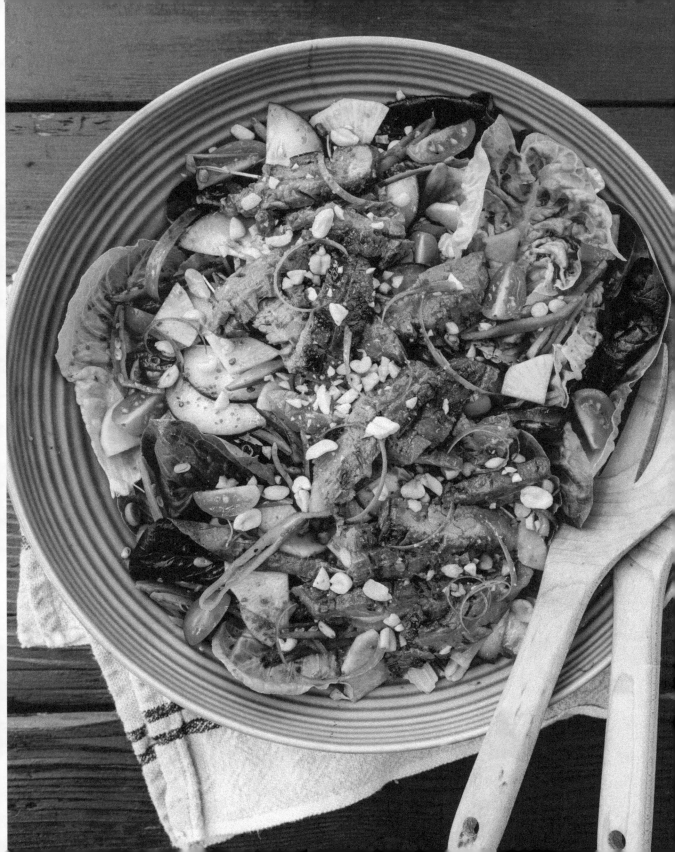

Miso-Marinated Flank Steak, Pickled Radishes, and Cucumber Salad
with Chile Oil and Crushed Peanuts

As the saying goes, if we're guaranteed anything in life, it's change. As a former vegetarian, I have to laugh at how much I love this salad. The steak, marinated in miso paste, garlic, and chiles, plays a major role. However, that's not to say you couldn't successfully swap the steak for a block of tofu. Either way, if you have the time, try to plan ahead for an overnight marinade for the deepest flavor. And consider using the chile oil with reckless abandon. It's not overly spicy, and it pulls the ingredients together just right.

Combine the tamari or soy sauce, rice vinegar, miso paste, garlic, grapeseed oil, and 1 teaspoon of the chile flakes in a large, sealable dish. Reserve a quarter of the marinade in a separate container in the refrigerator. Lightly score the steak, place it in the first dish, and turn to coat evenly. Cover tightly, and marinate for at least 4 hours, preferably overnight. Remove the steak from the refrigerator 30 minutes before grilling.

Preheat your grill (or heavy cast-iron pan, if cooking indoors) to medium-high. Cook the steak for 1 to 2 minutes per side to get a good sear. Lower the heat to medium, and transfer the meat to a cooler part of the grill for a couple more minutes per side, or until the internal temperature reaches 140° to 145°F (medium-rare). If cooking indoors, reduce the heat to medium and allow the steak to cook for a couple more minutes or until the desired internal temperature is reached. Remove the steak from the heat, and spoon the reserved marinade over it. Allow the meat to rest for 10 minutes before thinly slicing at an angle against the grain.

Toss the lettuce, cucumber, peas, tomatoes, pickled radishes, and scallions with the desired amount of chile oil in a large bowl. Arrange on a large serving platter, lay the steak over the top, and garnish with additional scallions, peanuts, Maldon sea salt, and black pepper. Drizzle more chile oil over the top just before serving, if desired.

SERVES 4

- ½ cup tamari or soy sauce
- 2 teaspoons unseasoned rice vinegar
- 1½ tablespoons white miso paste
- 2 cloves garlic, finely diced
- 1 tablespoon grapeseed oil
- 1 tablespoon dried chile flakes, divided
- 1½ pounds flank steak
- 1 head butter lettuce or 3–4 Little Gems
- 2½ cups thinly sliced cucumber
- 2 cups thinly sliced (lengthwise) sugar snap peas
- 1 cup halved cherry tomatoes
- 1 cup Pickled Radishes (page 87)
- 5–6 scallions, thinly sliced lengthwise and then roughly chopped, plus extra for garnish
- 1 cup Chile Oil (page 88)
- ½ cup roughly chopped Roasted Peanuts (page 84)
- sea salt and freshly cracked black pepper, plus Maldon salt for finishing

Masala Chai Braised Pork
and Garlic Udon Salad

SERVES 4

3–4 pounds bone-in pork shoulder

2 tablespoons finely ground whole masala chai tea

3 tablespoons grapeseed oil, divided

10 cloves garlic, 4 smashed, 6 finely diced

2 cups coconut milk (full fat is best)

1 cup filtered water

8 ounces round udon noodles

4 cups cleaned and roughly chopped maitake or other meaty mushroom

4 cups roughly chopped arugula or other peppery green

1 cup roughly chopped scallions, plus extra for garnish

sea salt and freshly cracked black pepper

This recipe was inspired by the intensely fragrant, creamy tea popular across many parts of India and Africa. You probably know the word chai *means "tea." Masala chai, however, is loaded with warming spices such as green cardamom, cinnamon, fennel, ginger, black pepper, star anise, cloves, and sweet coriander. In this recipe, the masala chai is finely ground and used as a rub for the pork, which is then slowly braised in rich coconut milk and garlic. After a couple of hours, the meat falls off the bone and the braising liquid becomes the sauce for deeply flavored and intensely satisfying udon noodles.*

NOTE: *Look for whole masala chai tea and grind in either a spice grinder or with a mortar and pestle.*

Preheat the oven to 325°F. Rub the pork with the finely ground chai tea blend, and season with salt and pepper. In a Dutch oven or other large, heavy, ovenproof stockpot over medium-high heat, add 1 tablespoon of the grapeseed oil. Once the oil is shimmering, add the pork shoulder.

Allow the pork to cook, untouched, for about 1 minute per side, until a golden crust forms all around. Then add the smashed garlic cloves, coconut milk, and filtered water, and season the braising liquid with salt and pepper. Transfer to the oven and braise for about 2½ to 3 hours, or until the meat falls off the bone and registers at least 145°F. Remove from the oven, and allow to cool slightly.

Cook the noodles according to the package instructions. Rinse with cold water, and set aside. When ready to assemble the salad, run hot water over the noodles to warm them through.

In a large skillet over medium-high heat, add the remaining 2 tablespoons of grapeseed oil. Once the oil is shimmering, add the mushrooms, and cook for about 4 to 5 minutes, or until they begin to turn golden on the edges. Turn off the heat, add the arugula and the finely diced garlic, and season with salt and pepper. Toss until the arugula is just wilted, about 1 minute, and keep warm in the pan.

This salad is great served warm or at room temperature. To assemble, shred the pork, and reserve the braising liquid. On a large serving platter or in individual bowls, place the pork, noodles, mushroom and arugula mixture, and scallions. Drizzle with the desired amount of braising liquid, and season with salt and pepper. Toss completely, and garnish with extra scallions.

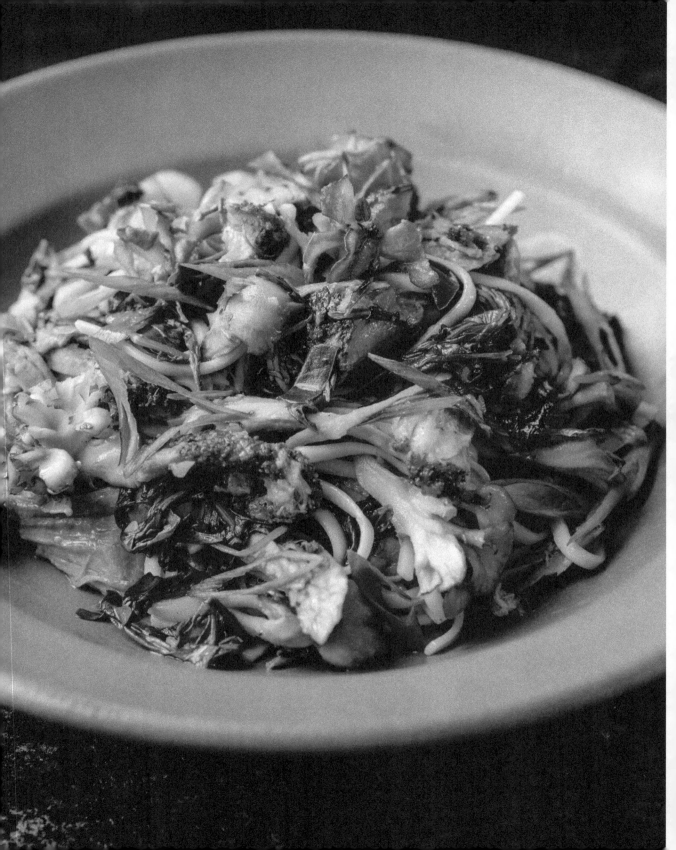

Star Anise Pork, Spicy Kimchi, and Soba Noodle Salad
with Caraway Oil

SERVES 4

8–10 star anise pods, finely ground

2½ teaspoons whole coriander, toasted and finely ground

3 cloves garlic, finely diced

3 tablespoons maple syrup, grade B, divided

2 tablespoons grapeseed oil, divided

1 (8-ounce) package buckwheat soba noodles

1–1½ pounds pork tenderloin, silver skin and surface fat removed

4 cups baby bok choy, thinly sliced into ¼-inch strips

1½ cups thinly sliced red bell pepper, julienned

2 cups roughly chopped Spicy Kimchi (page 90)

1 cup Caraway Oil (page 88)

1 cup Roasted Peanuts (page 84)

sea salt and freshly cracked black pepper, plus Maldon sea salt for finishing

During my undergraduate studies, I went through a phase in which I ate pot stickers almost every day. Not my proudest moments, but I was fascinated by the amount of flavor packed into those little dough pouches. This dish is inspired by the many combinations I've tried over the years. It's bold and spicy, slightly sweet, and a go-to favorite in my house. It's worth seeking out 100 percent buckwheat soba noodles for the richest flavor (especially if you've gone gluten-free).

Combine the ground star anise and coriander with the garlic, 2 tablespoons of the maple syrup, 1 tablespoon of the grapeseed oil, sea salt, and black pepper in a medium, sealable dish. Toss the tenderloin in the mixture until evenly coated. Cover tightly, and allow to marinate in the refrigerator for at least 2 hours, preferably overnight.

Cook the soba noodles according to the package instructions. Drain, rinse with cold water, and set aside until ready to assemble the salad.

Allow the tenderloin to sit at room temperature for 30 minutes. Preheat the oven to 400°F. Add the remaining 1 tablespoon of grapeseed oil to a large cast-iron skillet over medium heat. Once the oil is shimmering, add the tenderloin. Cook for 4 to 5 minutes on one side, or until a golden crust forms. Reduce the heat if the pork starts to blacken (the maple syrup can easily burn).

Turn the tenderloin over, and place the skillet in the oven for another 15 minutes, or until the internal temperature of the pork registers at least 145°F (medium rare). Remove from the skillet, drizzle with the remaining 1 tablespoon of maple syrup, and allow to rest for 10 minutes before slicing into thin medallions.

Toss the pork, bok choy, red pepper, kimchi, and noodles with the desired amount of caraway oil in a large serving bowl. Garnish with peanuts, Maldon sea salt, and black pepper before serving. Serve extra caraway oil on the side.

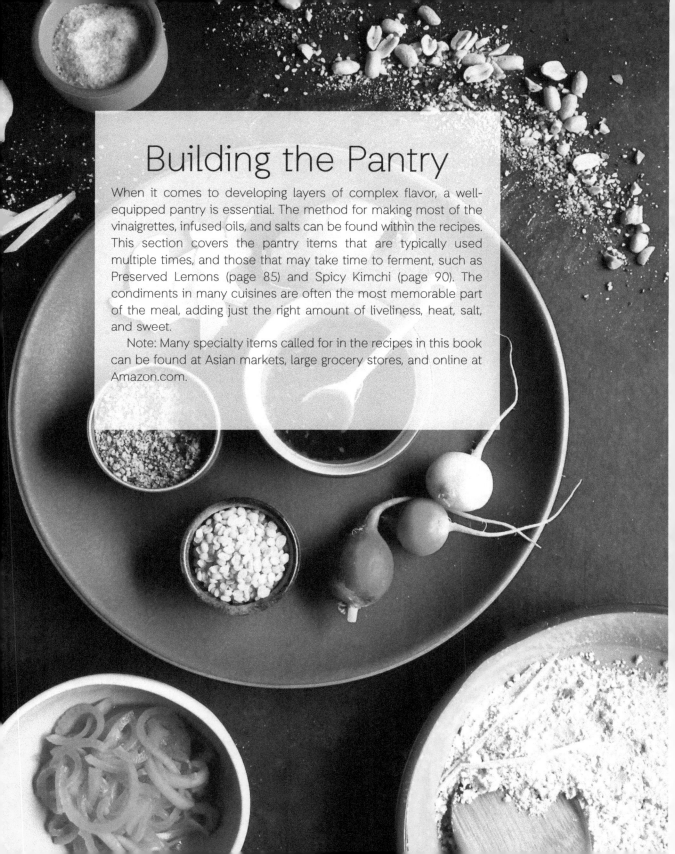

Building the Pantry

When it comes to developing layers of complex flavor, a well-equipped pantry is essential. The method for making most of the vinaigrettes, infused oils, and salts can be found within the recipes. This section covers the pantry items that are typically used multiple times, and those that may take time to ferment, such as Preserved Lemons (page 85) and Spicy Kimchi (page 90). The condiments in many cuisines are often the most memorable part of the meal, adding just the right amount of liveliness, heat, salt, and sweet.

Note: Many specialty items called for in the recipes in this book can be found at Asian markets, large grocery stores, and online at Amazon.com.

A NOTE ON SALT

As salt is the single most important element to make savory food shine, salt measurements are purposely not included because it is such a personal seasoning. (Because pepper is also a personal seasoning, measurements are not given for it, either.) Different types of salt vary in salinity, and I find that Himalayan pink salt works well in salads. Hand-mined, it contains the full spectrum of all 84 minerals, assists with electrolyte balance and nutrient absorption, and is one of the purest forms of salt available. Unrefined sea salt is a good substitution.

Many of the recipes in this book call for finishing salt, which provides a unique, crunchy texture and another layer of seasoning. My go-to is Maldon sea salt, for its burst of clean flavor that quickly dissolves on the tongue. Tamari, miso paste, and fish sauce also bring salty notes to these recipes. For the fish sauce, I recommend Red Boat 40°N.

INCORPORATING ACID

This refers to the characteristic sour flavor that provides brightness and is second in line of importance, next to salt, for balancing savory food. Citrus and vinegar are the two most commonly used acids in this book. Umeboshi plum vinegar, a brilliant magenta derivative of the pickling of umeboshi plums and red shiso leaf, and coconut vinegar, produced from the sap of coconut blossoms, are unique. They can both be purchased at most large grocery stores, or online at Amazon.com.

CHOOSING OILS

In my kitchen, I use a wide variety of oils and fats. Some are great for cooking while others are best in vinaigrettes. Two primary oils are used in this book: 1) organic, cold-pressed, extra virgin olive oil, and 2) organic, unrefined, hexane-free grapeseed oil. Olive oil has been a staple in the Mediterranean diet since as early as sixth century BC. Grapeseed oil, pressed from

the seeds of grapes, has been around for thousands of years as a health-promoting oil, as well. It has come under some recent scrutiny for its high polyunsaturated fat (PUFA) content and modern extraction by hexane, a hydrocarbon vapor derived from crude oil. The key is to choose a high-quality, unrefined oil, use it in moderation, and balance it with other fats.

Grapeseed oil has a neutral flavor, allowing the aromatics in these recipes to really shine. It also has a high smoke point, and can be used for numerous cooking methods. Olive oil is best when used raw, as in a vinaigrette, or when cooking at low temperatures to avoid oxidation.

Other good options to consider are organic, unrefined coconut oil, organic ghee (clarified butter), and organic, unrefined, cold-pressed avocado oil.

USING GRADE B MAPLE SYRUP

High in key minerals, such as zinc and manganese, maple syrup is my sweetener of choice. It also ranks extremely low on the glycemic index, and grade B is derived from sap harvested later in the season, producing a more intense flavor and color. Keep in mind that there are many artificial maple syrups on the market today, so look for a pure, organic maple syrup. It may cost more, but a little goes a long way.

INTEGRATING WHOLE SPICES AND CHILES

Fragrant, sweet, and peppery, whole spices each have their own characteristics. They add intense depth and a multitude of health benefits to food. Many of the recipes call for whole spices, which are then dry-toasted because they last longer and taste better than their pre-ground counterparts. Toasting whole spices also offers some control over the desired flavor outcome, makes them easier to grind, and releases aromatics that add complexity.

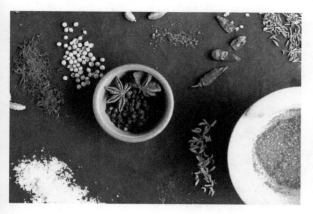

Chiles also have their own characteristics and are not only prized in the cuisine of Myanmar, but around the globe. Some offer acute heat, like the Thai bird chile used in Turkey Larb Salad (page 70). Others are milder, like the Japanese shishito pepper in French Lentil and Poached Egg Salad (page 40). After I played around with multiple chiles, Korean gochugaru chile rose to the top for the majority of the recipes in this book. This coarse, sun-dried chile flake has a stunning crimson color and a unique balance of sweet, spicy, and earthy notes.

GOCHUGARU CHILE

When purchasing this chile, know that *maewoon gochugaru* is very spicy while *deol maewoon gochugaru* is a milder version. Also, gochugaru can be easily confused with gochujang, a strong fermented Korean condiment made from red chile flakes, glutinous rice, fermented soybeans, and salt.

Recipes

Sticky Rice Powder

The purpose of sticky rice powder, or koa kore, is typically three-fold: 1) to add texture and a nutty, smoky flavor to salads, 2) to function as a thickening agent, and 3) for dipping unripe fruit, like green mango and guava, in Lao cuisine. While there may be temptation to skip this simple ingredient, it adds an undeniable complexity and authenticity.

YIELD: ABOUT 1 CUP

1 cup uncooked short-grain rice

1 lemongrass stalk, roughly chopped and crushed (optional)

Place a heavy skillet, like a cast-iron pan or wok, over medium heat, and add the rice. Toast for about 5 minutes, stirring occasionally with a wooden spoon. If using lemongrass, add it to the skillet with the rice, and toast for another 3 to 5 minutes, or until a uniform golden color is achieved. For a smokier flavor, cook the mixture for a few minutes longer, or until the rice reaches a light gray color.

Allow the rice to completely cool before grinding it to a fine powder in a spice grinder. Transfer to an airtight glass container, and store in a dark place for up to a month.

Toasted Chickpea Flour

A quintessential pantry staple in Burmese cuisine, chickpea flour, also known as gram or besan flour, is a gluten-free, protein-dense ingredient. When slowly toasted in a heavy cast-iron skillet, it morphs into a unique condiment that adds irrefutable texture and depth of flavor. Most Asian grocers, health food stores, and specialty food stores carry chickpea flour.

YIELD: 1 CUP
1 cup chickpea flour

Place a cast-iron or other heavy skillet over medium-high heat. Add the flour, and use a wooden spoon to stir occasionally until the flour begins to turn a light golden color. Lower the heat to medium, and continue to stir, exposing all the flour to the hot surface for an even toast.

After about 10 minutes, remove from the heat, continuing to stir occasionally until the skillet cools. You'll know the flour is properly toasted when it reaches a golden color and is aromatic. Transfer to a large plate, spreading out the flour to cool completely. Store in a glass jar at room temperature for up to a month.

Roasted Peanuts

My little boy carries a small mason jar of these peanuts around with him sometimes. They're a humble and satisfying way to incorporate texture and roasted flavor in many recipes. To him, at least, they're also the perfect snack.

YIELD: 1 CUP
1 cup whole raw peanuts

Place a cast-iron or other heavy skillet over medium heat, and add the peanuts. Stir them often with a wooden spoon to prevent burning. The end result should be an amber color that occurs gradually, after about 4 to 5 minutes. Once that is achieved, turn off the heat, stirring occasionally for another minute.

Transfer to a large plate, spreading the peanuts out to cool. Once they're cool, chop by hand or pulse in a food processor until you have some coarsely chopped pieces along with some powder. Transfer to a glass jar, and store in the refrigerator for up to a month.

Dukkah

Derived from the Arabic word dakka, *which means "to crush," dukkah (DOO-kah) is a versatile, and nutrient-dense Egyptian spice blend traditionally consisting of crushed nuts, seeds, and fresh spices. As is true of other regional spice blends, recipes vary across the globe. Nuts provide a good base and there are few limitations to what goes in next. Have fun creating your own blend.*

NOTE: *Any leftover is great as a rub for meat or fish, or as a garnish for soups or vegetables.*

YIELD: ABOUT 1¼ CUPS

¼ cup raw hazelnuts

¼ cup shelled raw pistachios

¼ cup raw sesame seeds

2 tablespoons raw, shelled sunflower seeds

2 tablespoons chia seeds

1 tablespoon whole cumin seeds

2 teaspoons whole coriander seeds

2 teaspoons whole fennel seeds

2 tablespoons unsweetened shredded coconut

½ teaspoon dried chile flakes (optional)

sea salt and freshly cracked black pepper

Toast the hazelnuts, pistachios, sesame seeds, sunflower seeds, chia seeds, cumin, coriander, fennel seeds, and coconut in separate batches in a dry skillet over medium heat, stirring occasionally, until light golden and fragrant. Each batch should take about 1 to 2 minutes. Set aside to cool.

The traditional method involves crushing the ingredients by hand with a mortar and pestle. If you have the time and inclination, this produces a beautiful, rustic result. Otherwise, combine all the toasted ingredients along with the chile flakes, if using, and salt and pepper in a food processor, and pulse until the mixture is coarsely ground. Take care not to overmix. The oils in the seeds and nuts are released when crushed by hand or processed. Too much friction will create a paste instead of the dry and crumbly result you want. Transfer to a glass jar, and refrigerate for up to a month.

Preserved Lemons

One of my favorite weekend morning rituals is to skim through my cookbooks while sipping coffee. I'm effortlessly transported to any part of the world via food. Middle Eastern flavors speak loudly to me on those lazy mornings. This recipe requires some advanced planning and patience, but the result is well worth the wait.

NOTE: *Meyer lemon is ideal, but the less sweet Eureka lemon, the variety most commonly found in grocery stores, will also work.*

YIELD: ABOUT 4 CUPS

10 medium lemons, rinsed and scrubbed well, plus 1 or 2 extra just for their juice

1 cup sea salt or kosher salt

Remove any tough stems from the lemons, and cut all the way through each lemon about ¼ to ½ inch from the tip. Then slice each lemon in half lengthwise, leaving it attached at the base. Make another cut as if you were going to slice it into quarters, but leave it connected. This allows the salt to permeate the lemon uniformly.

Generously sprinkle each lemon with salt on the inside and on the skin. Pack the lemons in a sterilized quart glass jar, pressing them down to eliminate air and to release their juices. If the lemons are not submerged in juice, add the juice of a couple more lemons until they are completely covered. Finish with a tablespoon of salt on the top, and seal the jar tightly.

Allow the lemons to sit on the counter at room temperature, out of the sun, for a few days, turning the jar upside down a couple times per day. Then transfer the jar to the refrigerator for at least 2 weeks, preferably for a minimum of a month, turning it upside down every couple of days. You'll know the lemons are ready when the rinds are soft.

To use, remove the amount of lemon you need, and rinse thoroughly under cold water. Slice the skin away from the pulp, removing any seeds and white pith, and discard. The preserved rind is then ready to use, so simply follow the recipe directions from there. Preserved lemons may be stored in the refrigerator for up to 6 months.

Crunchy Roasted Split Mung Dal

Small, green, and nutrient dense, the mung bean is a legume native to India. In fact, it has been considered one of the most cherished foods in the traditional Indian Ayurvedic diet for thousands of years. When skinned and split, the army green exterior gives way to a yellow, antioxidant-rich interior. Instead of using fried beans, common to most Burmese tea leaf salads, this recipe calls for slow roasting, to create that same addictive crunch.

NOTE: *Split mung dal (also called moong dal) can be found at many large grocery stores in the international or bulk section and online at Amazon.com. If you're unable to find these beans, yellow split peas are a good substitute. Just simmer them for an additional 5 minutes before roasting.*

YIELD: ABOUT 2 CUPS

2 cups dried split mung dal, rinsed and picked through for debris

3 tablespoons grapeseed oil

sea salt

Preheat the oven to 400°F. In a medium saucepan, add the mung dal and enough filtered water to cover the beans by at least 2 inches. Bring to a boil, and reduce the heat to medium-low. Simmer for 10 to 12 minutes, stirring occasionally.

Drain the beans, and dry them well between two clean kitchen towels. In a medium bowl, toss them with the grapeseed oil and sea salt until well coated. Arrange in an even layer on two parchment-lined baking sheets, and place on the middle racks of the oven. Roast for 10 minutes. Stir, and roast for another 10 to 15 minutes, or until crunchy and beginning to turn golden on the edges.

Allow the roasted mung dal to cool completely before transferring to a glass container. The beans are best used immediately, but they should remain crunchy for up to 5 days if stored in an airtight container at room temperature.

Pickled Red Onion

This is a quick pickle using tangy umeboshi plum vinegar, which imparts a brilliant hue of fuchsia. The pickle is great with everything from salads to burgers.

YIELD: ABOUT 1 CUP

1 medium red onion, halved and thinly sliced

½ cup umeboshi plum vinegar

½ cup filtered water

In a clean glass jar, combine the onion and vinegar with the filtered water. The onion should be completely submerged in the brining liquid. If it's not, add a little more filtered water. Cover and gently shake until well combined.

Allow to sit at room temperature for 4 to 5 hours, or until a bright pink color develops and the onion begins to soften. Refrigerate and use within a couple weeks. Umeboshi plum vinegar is quite salty, so if the onion becomes too strong, quickly rinse it before adding it to your dish.

Pickled Radishes

A crisp radish, sprinkled with flaky sea salt, is hard to beat. When the radish is pickled, however, the sharp, peppery notes become nuanced, allowing the inherent sweetness to come to the forefront. This quick pickle recipe intentionally creates a large batch, allowing leftovers for everything from creamy scrambled eggs to sandwiches and salads.

NOTE: *About 2 bunches of red radishes may be substituted. Just rinse and thinly slice them before tossing with salt.*

YIELD: ABOUT 3½ CUPS

2 medium watermelon radishes, peeled, quartered, and thinly sliced

1 (6-inch) daikon radish, peeled, quartered, and thinly sliced

generous pinch of sea salt

1 cup unseasoned rice vinegar

½ cup umeboshi plum vinegar

1 teaspoon whole black peppercorns

In a medium bowl, toss the radishes with the sea salt, and transfer them to a quart, wide-mouth glass jar. Add both vinegars and the peppercorns, and fill the remainder of the jar with filtered water. Cover and gently shake to combine the brine. Leave at room temperature for 1 to 2 days, then transfer to the refrigerator for up to 3 weeks.

Pickled Ginger

Most of the pickled ginger (gari) found at sushi restaurants is from China or Japan and contains food coloring to achieve that rosy hue. Brined in rice vinegar and umeboshi plum vinegar, this ultra-fresh recipe imparts that same hue without added chemicals. Young ginger is a good choice if you can find it.

NOTE: *A wine-based vinegar made from fruit such as fig or Muscat grape can be substituted for the umeboshi plum vinegar. Rearrange the ratio to ½ cup fruit vinegar and ½ cup rice vinegar, and start with a teaspoon or two of maple syrup, adjusting to your liking from there.*

YIELD: ABOUT 1 CUP

1 cup shaved young (or mature) ginger

¼ cup umeboshi plum vinegar

¾ cup unseasoned rice vinegar

1 tablespoon maple syrup, grade B

Bring a medium saucepan of water to a boil. Remove the skin from the ginger using the back of a spoon or a paring knife. Using a vegetable peeler or mandoline, shave the ginger into different sizes. Blanch the ginger in the boiling water for about 3 minutes to reduce the sharpness. Drain, and transfer the ginger to a medium bowl. Add the vinegars and maple syrup, stir to completely combine, then transfer to a glass jar. Place in the refrigerator, and use within a month.

Caraway Oil

Caraway is not actually a seed, but rather a dried fruit grown in many parts of Asia, Europe, North Africa, and North America. Used most commonly in rye bread, caraway has a sweet, nutty, anise-like flavor.

YIELD: ABOUT 1¼ CUPS

3 tablespoons whole caraway seeds, roughly ground

1 cup grapeseed oil

sea salt and freshly cracked black pepper

In a medium saucepan over medium heat, add the caraway seeds, and, stirring occasionally, toast for 1 minute, or until aromatic. Add the grapeseed oil, and bring to a boil over medium-high heat. Once boiling, turn off the heat, and season with salt and pepper.

Allow to cool before transferring to a glass container. Refrigerate for up to 2 weeks, and bring to room temperature before using.

Chile Oil

This is one of those pantry ingredients I don't know how I ever lived without. It's visually stunning with a deep ruby-red color, great on just about everything, and could not be easier to make. Gochugaru chile is recommended for this recipe, but Aleppo chile may be substituted.

YIELD: ABOUT 1 CUP

1 cup grapeseed oil

1 tablespoon chile flakes

pinch of sea salt

In a medium saucepan, heat the oil over medium-high heat, then add the chile flakes. Once boiling, turn off the heat and add the sea salt. Allow to cool, and transfer to a glass jar. It can be refrigerated for up to 2 weeks.

Crispy Shallots and Shallot Oil

If you love to multitask, this recipe will hit your sweet spot. In less than 15 minutes, you can create two deeply flavored pantry items that add immense flavor and texture. The key is to go slow to get a uniform golden color, and to infuse the oil with as much shallot flavor as possible.

NOTE: *Peanut oil is used in many Asian preparations, but I prefer grapeseed oil for its lower saturated fat content and neutral flavor.*

YIELD: ABOUT 1 CUP SHALLOT OIL; ABOUT 1½ CUPS CRISPY SHALLOTS

1 cup grapeseed oil

2–2½ cups thinly sliced shallots (about 5–6 large shallots)

sea salt

In a large skillet over medium-high heat, add the grapeseed oil. Once the oil is shimmering, add a test slice of shallot. If it begins to sizzle vigorously, carefully toss the remaining slices into the oil.

Stirring occasionally, allow the temperature to come back up until the sizzling begins again. Then lower the heat to medium, and cook for about 10 to 12 minutes, or until golden brown, stirring frequently. The shallots will shrink as they crisp.

Remove with a slotted spoon, and transfer the crispy shallots to a paper towel–lined plate to cool. Season with salt. Once cool, store in a glass container for up to 5 days. They may lose some of their crispness over time, but the flavor will still be excellent.

For the shallot oil, allow it to cool, then pass it through a fine-mesh strainer into a glass jar. If stored in a cool, dark spot, the oil will keep for a couple of weeks.

Crispy Garlic and Garlic Oil

In my opinion, this duo is a must for the tea leaf salad. Leaving some of the garlic slices intact while finely chopping others makes for an interesting texture.

YIELD: ABOUT 1 CUP GARLIC OIL; ABOUT ¼ CUP CRISPY GARLIC

1 cup grapeseed oil

¾ cup thinly sliced cloves garlic (about 15 cloves garlic)

sea salt

In a medium saucepan over medium-high heat, warm the oil until it begins to shimmer. Toss one garlic slice in. Once the garlic begins to sizzle, add the remainder, and allow the oil to come back to almost boiling. Reduce the heat to medium, shaking the pan occasionally to evenly crisp the garlic.

After 2 to 3 minutes, a light golden color will begin to develop. Once all the slices are uniformly golden, remove them with a slotted spoon, and drain on a paper towel–lined plate. Season with sea salt. Once cool, finely dice some of the slices, if desired.

For the garlic oil, allow it to cool, then pass it through a fine-mesh strainer into a glass jar. If stored in a cool, dark spot, the oil will be good for a couple of weeks.

Spicy Kimchi

I once heard a Korean woman poetically describe how chile peppers should "splash smoothly across the tongue." For kimchi, at least, I have to agree. Tolerably hot, with an earthy, fruity, and slightly smoky flavor, Korean red chile flakes, called gochugaru, are the star ingredient in this recipe. Aleppo chile is a good substitution, however. I included dried bonito flakes and, as a nod to my Hungarian roots, smoked paprika in this modern version.

NOTE: *Making kimchi from scratch requires some patience and time. It would be easy for me to say it is worth it. The real evidence came from watching several friends devour this kimchi, straight out of the jar, while standing over my kitchen sink.*

YIELD: ABOUT 4 CUPS

1 large Napa cabbage (about 5 pounds)

1 cup coarse sea salt or kosher salt, divided

7 cups filtered water, divided

1 tablespoon Sticky Rice Powder (page 83)

½ cup gochugaru chile pepper flakes

2 tablespoons dried bonito flakes

½ sheet dried untoasted seaweed (nori), roughly broken into pieces

2 tablespoons fish sauce

1 teaspoon smoked paprika

3 tablespoons grated ginger

4 cloves garlic, roughly chopped

1 tablespoon maple syrup, grade B

½ cup roughly chopped scallions

1 pound daikon radish, julienned (optional)

¼ cup julienned Asian pear, (optional)

sea salt and freshly cracked black pepper

To prepare the cabbage, carefully cut it into quarters lengthwise ensuring the stem remains intact. Dissolve ½ cup of the coarse or kosher salt in a large bowl filled with 6 cups of the filtered water. Soak each quarter of the cabbage in the salted water individually, for about 1 to 2 minutes, before shaking the excess water back into the bowl.

Use the remaining ½ cup of salt to generously sprinkle over each cabbage quarter, beginning with the outer leaf and working inward. Place each quarter in another large bowl, and pour the water from the original salt bath over the top. Set aside for at least 5 hours, preferably 8 hours, or until the white leaves are soft.

Rinse thoroughly, removing the salt from each leaf, and drain well. Set aside while you make the kimchi mixture.

Place the sticky rice powder in a small saucepan with about ½ cup of the filtered water, and bring to a boil. This will happen quickly. Once boiling, lower the heat and, stirring occasionally, simmer until a thick paste is reached, about 1 to 2 minutes. Remove the saucepan from the heat, and allow to cool.

Add the cooled rice powder paste along with the chile pepper flakes, dried bonito flakes, nori, fish sauce, paprika, ginger, garlic, and maple syrup to a food processor. Add the remaining ½ cup of the filtered water, and pulse until combined, scraping down the sides as you go. The mixture should be a little chunky. Transfer to a large bowl, and toss with the scallions and, if using, the radish and pear. Taste for salt, and adjust if needed. The mixture should be overly salty for the best finished result.

Cut off the tough stem of each drained cabbage quarter, and discard. Spread the rice powder mixture evenly over each quarter, leaf by leaf. Once complete, roll up each quarter from the outside in. Place all four quarters in a sterilized quart jar, pressing down on the bundles to remove any excess air. Any extra can be placed in a smaller, sterilized jar using the same process.

Allow the kimchi to sit at room temperature for at least 2 to 3 days. After two days, gently loosen the lid to allow some pressure to release. Tighten the lid again, and allow to sit out another day, if possible, before transferring to the refrigerator. For best results, allow to mature for at least another 2 weeks in the refrigerator, and use within a month.

Transformative Foods

Most of us know by now that superfoods, typically fruits and vegetables, are bursting with antioxidants, phytonutrients, fiber, and other macro- and micro-nutrients. These high-performance foods have the power to dramatically change our internal landscape and even protect our DNA from damage. With the ability to affect change in such a profound way, these foods could be considered transformative. Food is information for the body, after all. And each of us carries a unique biochemical makeup that is influenced by the nutrients we consume, or don't consume.

Used throughout this book, the following transformative foods are nutrient-rich and they assist in the creation of an environment where health is a likely outcome when eaten on a regular basis. Remember to choose the freshest organic food whenever possible.

AVOCADO: Consisting primarily of monounsaturated fats (like those found in olive oil and nuts), avocados are creamy and nutrient-dense food. Beneficial elements include folate, phytonutrients, and vitamins E and K.

BEETS: With unique phytonutrient pigments, beets are antioxidant workhorses with an especially rich folate (B9) content, essential for healthy tissue growth, DNA repair, and heart health. Beet greens provide a higher nutrient-density than the roots themselves, offering more iron than spinach, and notable amounts of zinc, vitamins A and C, and calcium.

BLACK GARLIC: Not entirely mainstream yet, the antioxidant-rich fermented black garlic brings on a complex sweet-sour flavor (reminiscent of molasses, balsamic vinegar, tamarind, or dried prunes) and a soft, chewy texture known for providing significant free-radical protection in the body.

One of my favorite restaurants in San Francisco, Bar Tartine, makes their own black garlic. Here's their method, if you're feeling adventurous:

Wrap garlic heads in plastic wrap to trap the humidity and keep the garlic moist. Next, wrap the heads in several layers of aluminum foil. Place in a dehydrator, at 130°F, and let sit until the heads are black and soft, about three weeks. You can also use a rice warmer or slow cooker, placed on the warm or low setting for about two weeks. Store in an airtight container, in the refrigerator, for up to six months. To use, peel the cloves and gently press out the garlic.

Black garlic can also be purchased at some specialty markets and online at www.blackgarliccity.com.

CITRUS: An example of everyday ingredients with health benefits, citrus is high in vitamins A and C, fiber, folate, calcium, and potassium, and is well known for its remarkable ability to assist in the body's natural detoxification process.

COCONUT: Not technically a nut, but rather a drupe (stone fruit), coconuts are loaded with lauric acid, which is known to increase immunity and destroy harmful pathogens. They are also high in fiber, naturally occurring electrolytes, and healthy fatty acids that the body metabolizes quickly.

CRUCIFEROUS (BRASSICA) VEGETABLES: Broccoli, cabbage, kale, boy choy, collard greens, turnips, kohlrabi, mustard greens, and Brussels sprouts are all cruciferous vegetables. When each of these plants goes to seed and flower, a cross-like design emerges. This is where the name crucifer, or "cross-bearer" in Latin, came to be.

Known for their fierce ability to ward off and even halt some diseases, brassicas contain unique sulfur compounds and phytochemicals in addition to an impressive fiber, vitamin, and mineral content. Plus, their nooks are great for absorbing flavor.

FERMENTS: Fermentation is an ancient practice, serving primarily as a means to preserve and liberate nutrients and medicinal properties in certain foods.

When carbohydrates and sugars are converted into alcohol or acids, beneficial bacteria are fused into new enzyme-rich forms. These changes affect our gut microbiota, contributing to greater immunity, decreased inflammation and oxidative stress, and heightened positive mental health.

LEAFY GREENS & MICROGREENS: The fundamental building block for many salads, leafy greens provide more nutrients, calorie-for-calorie, than most other foods. Fiber, folate, carotenoids, iron, calcium, and vitamins A, B, C, E, and K can be found in everything from spinach to pea shoots.

Recent research found that microgreens, edible young greens harvested about two weeks after seeding, may provide four to six times more nutrients than the mature leaves of the same vegetable or herb plant.

LEGUMES: Among the most consumed foods in the world, lentils, peas, and beans have been a staple for thousands of years. They're cost-efficient, nutrient-rich, and a substantial source of protein, fiber, antioxidants, anti-carcinogens, phytochemicals, vitamins, and minerals. These little gems are often associated with reduced risk of many chronic diseases.

MISO PASTE: Miso is made by combining cooked soybeans with koji, cooked rice inoculated with a fermentation culture. It's basically a sweet mold that forms the foundation for many fermented products, including soy sauce, mirin, and rice vinegar. This process creates a paste that is especially nutrient-dense, full of live cultures, vitamins, and minerals, and is easily assimilated by the body. Miso is also high in linoleic acid, a polyunsaturated omega-6 fat, known for maintaining skin health and integrity.

NUTS: An ancient and modern staple, nuts have long been associated with increased cardiovascular health. Loaded with fiber, they also contain a wide range of vitamins, antioxidants, essential fatty acids, and phytochemicals. Recent studies suggest the more nuts people consume, the greater their chances of avoiding most major diseases, especially heart disease and stroke.

SEAWEED: One of the world's most nutritious and sustainable plants, seaweed absorbs phosphorous, nitrogen, and carbon dioxide directly from the sea and grows at an impressive rate (9–12 feet in as little as three months!). Seaweed is one of the richest sources of iodine, an essential trace mineral often deficient in the modern diet; it's also rich in amino acids, antioxidants, and enzymes. The bioactive nutrients in seaweed impact the body at the cellular level, resulting in significant benefit to the skin, nails, and hair.

SEEDS: Used abundantly throughout this book, seeds are tiny, nutritious treasures. They're a fiber-rich way to incorporate a balance of omega-3 and omega-6 fatty acids, especially when several varieties are consumed together.

TAMARIND: The tamarind tree can often be found in tropical climates, particularly in parts of South Asia and Mexico. A member of the legume family, the pod-encased fruit was traditionally used in Ayurvedic medicine to alleviate digestive issues. The potent, super-sour flesh has been touted to promote heart health, lower cholesterol, and provide an impressive amount of vitamin C.

WILD MUSHROOMS: There are tens of thousands of species of mushroom-forming fungi, of which we only know about 10–15 percent. Incorporating a variety of wild mushrooms builds on texture and flavor. An excellent source of antioxidants, wild mushrooms also contain L-ergothioneine (ERGO), a potent sulfur-containing antioxidant. In fact, some scientists now refer to ERGO as the "master antioxidant," which plays a major role in protecting DNA from oxidative damage.

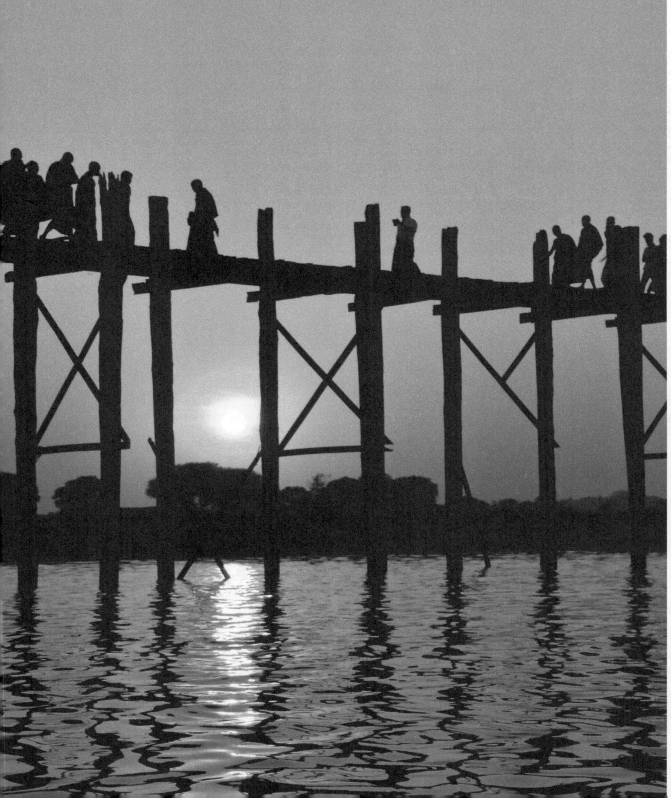

Conversions

VOLUME CONVERSIONS

U.S.	U.S. EQUIVALENT	METRIC
1 tablespoon (3 teaspoons)	½ fluid ounce	15 milliliters
¼ cup	2 fluid ounces	60 milliliters
⅓ cup	3 fluid ounces	90 milliliters
½ cup	4 fluid ounces	120 milliliters
⅔ cup	5 fluid ounces	150 milliliters
¾ cup	6 fluid ounces	180 milliliters
1 cup	8 fluid ounces	240 milliliters
2 cups	16 fluid ounces	480 milliliters

WEIGHT CONVERSIONS

U.S.	METRIC
½ ounce	15 grams
1 ounce	30 grams
2 ounces	60 grams
¼ pound	115 grams
⅓ pound	150 grams
½ pound	225 grams
¾ pound	350 grams
1 pound	450 grams

TEMPERATURE CONVERSIONS

FAHRENHEIT (°F)	CELSIUS (°C)
70°F	20°C
100°F	40°C
120°F	50°C
130°F	55°C
140°F	60°C
150°F	65°C
160°F	70°C
170°F	75°C
180°F	80°C
190°F	90°C
200°F	95°C
220°F	105°C
240°F	115°C
260°F	125°C
280°F	140°C
300°F	150°C
325°F	165°C
350°F	175°C
375°F	190°C
400°F	200°C
425°F	220°C
450°F	230°C

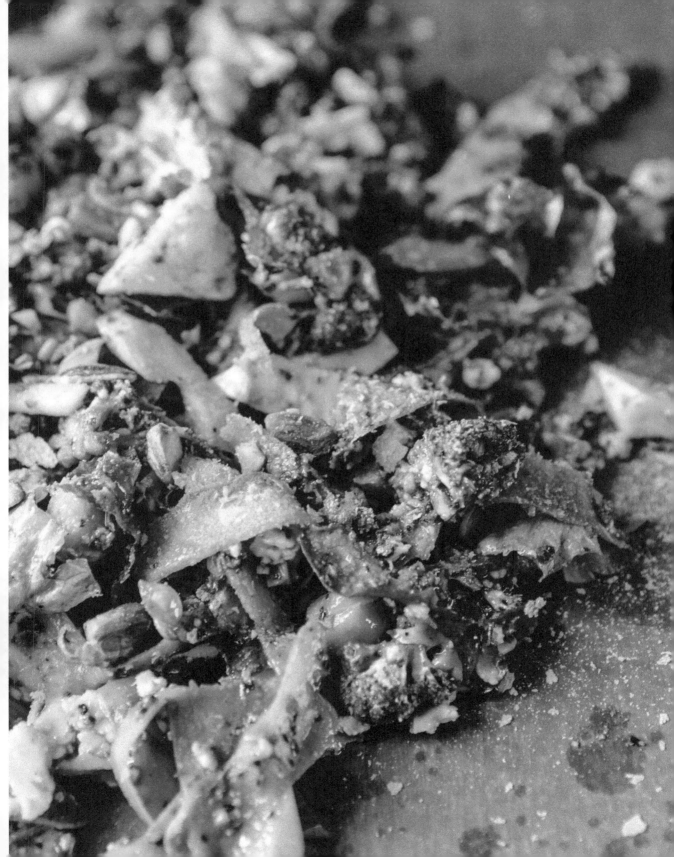

Bibliography

Balla, Nicholaus and Cortney Burns. *Bar Tartine: Techniques and Recipes*. (San Francisco, CA: Chronicle Books, 2014) 39.

Bloomberg Business. "Burma and Myanmar: From Junta Repression to Luxury Tourism." Accessed December 23, 2015. www.bloomberg.com/news/articles/2015-12-23/burma-and-myanmar-from-junta-repression-to-luxury-tourism.

Beelman, Robert. "Ergothioneine in Mushrooms— Nature's Best Source of a New Human Vitamin?" (presentation at annual Mushroom Industry Conference, Penn State University, University Park, PA, July 11–13, 2006).

The Chopra Center. "The Six Tastes." Accessed January 11, 2015. http://www.chopra.com/the-six-tastes.
Dornenburg, Andrew and Karen Page. *Culinary Artistry*. (Hoboken, NJ: Wiley Publishing, 1996) 37–72.

Duguid, Naomi. *Burma: Rivers of Flavor*. (New York: Artisan, 2012) 1–73, 97, 192, 306–321.

Fisher, M.F.K. *The Art of Eating*. (Hoboken, NJ: Wiley Publishing, 2004) 57–74, 350.

Katz, Sandor Ellix. *The Art of Fermentation: An In-Depth Exploration of Essential Concepts and Processes from around the World*. (White River Junction, VT: Chelsea Green Publishing, 2012) 18–35, 95–144.

Kelly, Laura. "Culinary History Mystery #4: The Origins of Tea in Burma." Last modified May 4, 2011. www.silkroadgourmet.com/the-origins-of-tea-in-burma.

Page, Karen and Andrew Dornenburg. *The Flavor Bible*. (New York: Little, Brown and Company, Hachette Book Group, 2011) 1–22, 51, 149, 188, 223, 275–297.

Selhub E. M., A. C. Logan, and A. C. Bested. "Fermented Foods, Microbiota, and Mental Health: Ancient Practice Meets Nutritional Psychiatry." NCBI (2014). Accessed February 23, 2016. www.ncbi.nlm.nih.gov/pubmed/24422720.

Thwe, Pascal Khoo. *From the Land of Green Ghosts: A Burmese Odyssey*. (New York: Harper Perennial, 2003) xiii–43

Tearroir. "Get High on Tea: Altitude's Effect on Tea." Last modified September 14, 2012. http://tearroir.com/premium-loose-leaf-teas/high-atltitude-tea-getting-high-on-tea#.Vtibg5MrLNB.

The Wall Street Journal. "People Who Taste Too Much." Last modified March 19, 2013. www.wsj.com/articles/SB10001424127887324392804578362833147151480

The Wine Economist. "Sababay Wines of Bali: New Latitudes, New Flavors, New Frontiers." Last modified August 26, 2014. http://wineeconomist.com/2014/08/26/sababay.

Recipe Index

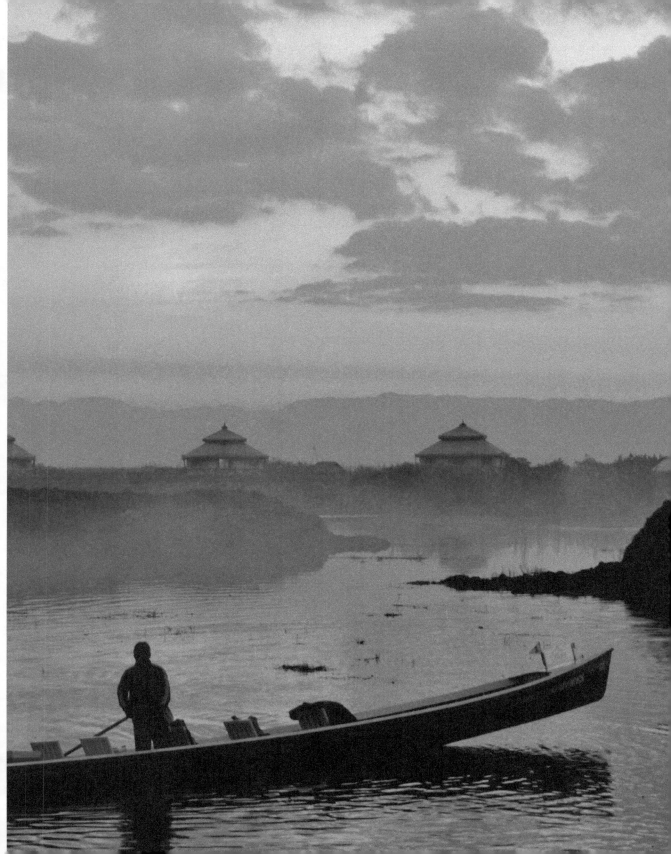

Acknowledgments

Like most things in life, this book is a collective effort. So many people rallied around me with patience, persistence, excitement, and creativity to pull this off. I'd first like to express gratitude to the four people whose support ultimately made this project possible:

To Corbin and Fletcher, thank you for taking care of each other while I worked long hours, for your willingness to taste everything (who knew a little boy could love nutritional yeast so much?), and for providing space and support for this book to come to life. Also, for taking my obsessive-compulsiveness with a grain of salt. This book is really yours.

And to my parents, who always picked up the phone and provided unconditional love, advice, and support during the unfolding of this book. Most important, for introducing me to the world of food at such an early age.

To Kimberley Hasselbrink, for not only creating lovely images, but for becoming a friend to laugh (and drink end-of-shoot wine) with along the way. Thanks for sharing your incredible talent, playing prop stylist, food stylist, assistant, and dishwasher when necessary. And for breaking me out of my comfort zone, often.

To the wonderful team at Ulysses Press, especially Alice Riegert and Keith Riegert. Thank you for giving me this opportunity. Your patience, guidance, and desire to create an inspiring book never wavered. Most of all, thank you for believing in me.

A special thanks to Susan Lang, for combing through the many tangles.

To the entire Howes and Penman family, you have supported my dreams for years, cheering me on from the sidelines. Your faith often pulled me through, and I thank you for that colossal gift.

To Adam and Genevieve Weiner, for sharing their Sonoma home as a writer's retreat and makeshift photo studio, despite the hilarious and ongoing garbage disposal/plumbing issues on my watch. You saved the day, so many times.

My dedicated testing community, with special thanks to Kirsten Prunty and Jeff and Kimbria Ralls, your invaluable feedback and recipe refinement provided the backbone for this book. I could not have done this without you. Thank you, thank you, thank you!

To Rebecca Katz, Melissa Lanz, Dianne Jacob, Sarah Forman, Nathan Lyon, Leslie Harlib, Devatara Holman, and everyone else who provided expert guidance along the way. I am forever grateful for each of you. Melissa, you couldn't have been more right: one recipe a day!

To Marion Montgomery, Amy Iftekhar, Nancy Williams, and Cindee Rood for the beautiful Myanmar images, stories, and willingness to share your firsthand adventures.

To Lauri Neidell, for helping me find my true north.

To my friends near and far, thank you for understanding when I was often too busy to get together but for offering encouragement and love, nonetheless. You know who you are, but a very heartfelt thanks to the following people:

Marta Corley, Alma Hunter, Janna Bennett, Lisa Shuster, Jamyn Peralta, Devorah Duemler, Carol Williams, Kristen Sperling, Jackie Reinhart, Micky Doner, Natalie Long, Lynn Yuster, Kory Johnston, Vanessa Seidler, Lisa Sullivan, Kirsten Prunty (again!), Sean and Bria Martin, and Tom Cebellero.

To Suresh, for that serendipitous conversation. I will always think of you with gratitude.

Finally, to the people of Myanmar, for creating thrilling food and inspiring continuous reinvention in us all.

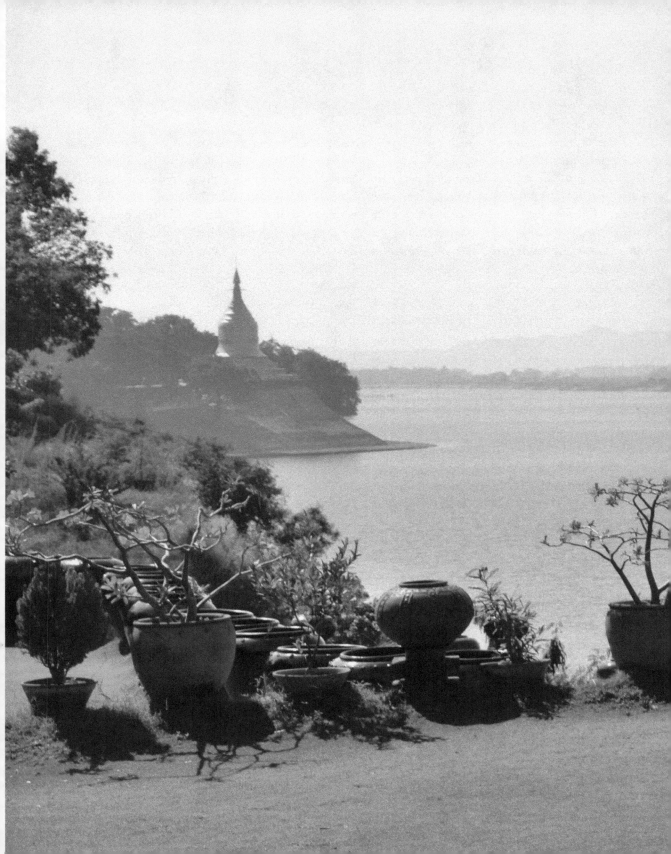

About the Author

ELIZABETH HOWES writes about food, culture, and travel. She is also a chef, recipe developer, and wellness consultant. Raised bi-coastally in a family full of inspired cooks and culinary entrepreneurs, the world of food became her home at an early age. When she moved to San Francisco, she used years of study and hands-on experimentation with various cooking techniques to develop her culinary style: highly creative, health-driven, and wildly flavorful food. Elizabeth has appeared on the Food Network, and in the James Beard Foundation's, *JBF Notes*. Her work has been featured on Shape.com, Edible Marin & Wine Country, Slow Food Marin, and Gojee.com, among others. She lives just outside of San Francisco with her son, who can't get enough white truffle oil, garden tomatoes, or turmeric.

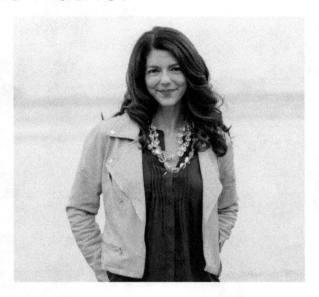

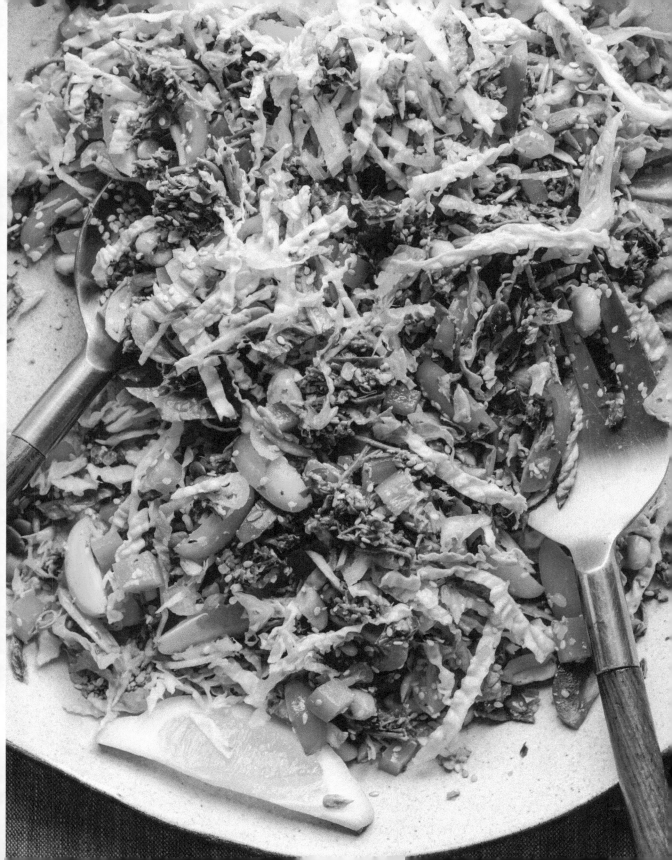

www.ingramcontent.com/pod-product-compliance
Lightning Source LLC
Chambersburg PA
CBHW060822190125
20459CB00007B/88